GOLDEN HOURS

Ignorance is no Longer a Bliss

Dr. N.K. Venkataramana

STARDOM BOOKS

www.StardomBooks.com

STARDOM BOOKS
112 Bordeaux Ct.
Coppell, TX 75019, USA

FIRST EDITION MARCH 2026

STARDOM BOOKS, LLC.
112 Bordeaux Ct. Coppell, TX 75019, USA

www.stardombooks.com

Stardom Books
United States and India

GOLDEN HOURS
Ignorance is no Longer a Bliss

Dr. N.K. Venkataramana

p. 153
cm. 13.5 X 21.5

Category : HEA039110 Health & Fitness : Diseases - Nervous System
(incl. Brain)
MED057000 Medical : Neuroscience
MED085010 Medical : Surgery - Neurosurgery

ISBN : 978-1-957456-86-7

Dedication

To all those generous minds who joined hands and
gave their whole hearted support to this life saving project.

Acknowledgments

First and foremost, my heartfelt gratitude to the Almighty for granting me the strength, commitment, insight, and zeal to undertake this endeavor, which has saved countless lives and brought immense satisfaction and fulfillment. It has been an inspiration and a profound learning experience of a lifetime.

I wish to express my sincere thanks to **Mr. Sridhar Raman** for his editorial contribution to the first draft. My deep gratitude also goes to **Capt. C. R. Gopinath**, Founder of Deccan Aviation, for his captivating and inspiring Foreword.

My sincere thanks to all my teachers, who have been my sources of knowledge, guidance, and wisdom, and for shaping me into a compassionate neurosurgeon and lifelong learner.

A project of this scale could never have been conceptualized or executed without the unwavering support of countless individuals and institutions. I have been fortunate to receive immense and timely help —financial, technical, intellectual, physical, moral, and social —at every critical juncture. Each time a crisis arose, a new avenue opened, reaffirming my faith in collective goodwill. Though it is impossible to name everyone individually, I express my deepest gratitude to each one of them from the bottom of my heart.

My heartfelt thanks to all the office staff, secretaries, doctors, paramedics, volunteers, drivers, social activists, and fellow NGOs who selflessly rendered their services and contributed to this mission.

My deepest appreciation goes to my wife and daughter, **Dr. Shobha Venkat** and **Dr. Bharggavi**, for their unconditional love, patience, and encouragement throughout this journey.

A special note of thanks to **Dr. Kamalesh** and **Mrs. Bharathi Kamalesh** for being a constant source of inspiration in documenting these experiences.

I am also deeply grateful to the **core team of trustees** for their faith in me and for their dedicated stewardship of the not-for-profit trust.

My sincere appreciation to the **Media, Police, Hospital authorities, Government officials,** and **educational institutions** for their collaboration and support.

Finally, my special thanks to the dedicated team at **Stardom Books** for shaping this book with such care and elegance.

Contents

Foreword

A Life of Purpose and Persistence : The Journey of
Dr. Venkataramana

— Capt. C R Gopinath

Founder of Deccan Aviation

Dr. N.K. Venkataramana, Founder Chairman of BRAINS super-specialty Hospital, Bangalore, is a man on a mission, driven by a profound sense of purpose and a missionary zeal. Cynics may call his indomitable pursuit of a world where no one dies for the want of urgent medical attention, a "mission impossible." History shows that those who change the world are dreamers with unshakeable purpose and courage of conviction. We all have heard about saints, visionaries and reformers in great detail.

Whether it is Mahatma Gandhi and Swami Vivekananda or great scientists such as Marie Curie and Albert Einstein, all of them remain connected by one common thread. They are united in a strong belief in their purpose. In times where people turn hateful and remain skeptical, it is this perseverance that drives them forward.

Such individuals do not succumb to despair when faced with setbacks or when circumstances spiral beyond their control. Instead, they throw themselves into action, fueled by dogged persistence, boundless energy, and an unshakable optimism. They refuse to lose hope, trusting that their efforts will, if not eradicate, at least mitigate suffering and pain.

It is this beacon of hope that sustains and propels them forward.

Dr. Venkataramana belongs to this rare class of individuals.

On one hand, he has delved deeply into the mysteries of the brain, dedicating himself to cutting-edge research and the creation of a state-of-the-art neuro care facility. On the other hand, he has committed his life to social service through the not-for-profit NGO, Comprehensive Trauma Consortium (CTC).

His vision is to aid trauma victims with timely medical assistance by establishing an integrated, competent system of air and ground ambulances that are connected by a seamless communication network.

This will make sure that patients reach hospitals within the critical "Golden Hour," a window in which timely medical intervention can save lives and prevent long-term disabilities.

The reality is stark: most trauma victims do not survive because they cannot access medical care within one to two hours of an accident, heart attack, or other emergencies. This is so particularly in remote areas.

A tragic irony exists in India: while hospitals offer insurance coverage for treatment post-admission, there is no universal coverage for air ambulance services. Air ambulances lack accessibility. They are available only to those that possess wealth. However, the situation is quite different in the US, Australia and Europe. These places have made these services affordable to the larger population by leveraging insurance models that are new, innovative and resourceful. India can follow suit by scaling insurance products at a larger level. This could aid access to air ambulances and turn a luxury into a service that can save lives.

I had the good fortune of meeting Dr Venkataramana two decades ago through a chance encounter. At the time, I was running the Deccan Helicopter Services from Jakkur Airfield. One night, I received an urgent call from a doctor at Manipal Hospital, requesting an emergency airlift for a young female doctor who had been severely injured in a bus accident on the Bangalore-Hyderabad highway.

I immediately contacted my colleague, Captain Jayanth Poovaiah, and asked him to get ready for an emergency flight.

The crew jumped into action and by 4 am had revamped the helicopter entirely. Stretchers were put into place, fuel was loaded and the medical team from Manipal soon departed.

The flight stretched 200 kilometers.

Post the hour-long journey, the team located the site of the accident, touched down in an adjacent field, and airlifted the injured woman.

Despite reaching Jakkur swiftly, it took another hour to transfer her to Manipal Hospital, where, tragically, she succumbed to her injuries upon arrival.

The following day, Dr. Venkataramana and his team visited us at Deccan to discuss ways to improve medical evacuations in the face of a plethora of infrastructural challenges—congested roads, lack of dedicated air ambulances, regulatory hurdles, and hospitals without helipads. These issues, and potential solutions, are explored in depth throughout this book.

Dr. Venkataramana houses a resilient spirit, he continues to produce new ideas despite limited resources and obstacles. As he so articulately states in the book:

"Despite having a relatively small vehicular population of four million, accidents in India claim around 90,000 lives annually. In comparison, developed nations with 140 million vehicles report only about 39,000 deaths.

The death rate per 1,000 vehicles in the U.S. is two, compared to a staggering 140 in India. This disparity can be attributed to deplorable road conditions, inadequate vehicle maintenance, unsafe driving practices, a flawed licensing system, lack of oversight, and more. However, there is no doubting the fact that most of these deaths could be prevented if only India had a robust Medical Emergency Response System, even half as efficient as the one I experienced in Germany."

It is easy to criticize and necessary to call out inefficiencies. However, what truly matters is taking action to address the challenges we face. Dr. Venkataramana has blazed a trail, illuminating the path forward for us all.

Preface

From solar-powered highway clinics and air ambulances to GPS-driven communication systems and robust networks of mobile ICUs, **Dr. N. K. Venkataramana, the Man of the Golden Hour,** has accomplished it all in his 30-year career dedicated to saving lives and alleviating human suffering.

This is the true story of an indomitable neurosurgeon who, stirred and shaken by a traumatic emergency room tragedy in his early years, battled daunting bureaucratic, logistic, and financial odds over decades to build systems and institutions that could respond with speed and compassion to human crises.

It is the story of an era that went from outdated pagers and faxes to futuristic smartphones and artificial intelligence, changing everything except the resolve of one man.

A moving saga of persistence and perseverance of a changemaker who has borne the cross of a pioneer, often at unbearable personal costs, with extraordinary grace and will to accomplish his mission of MERSY, or Mobile Emergency Response System.

Dr Venkataramana's first experience of how quickly and dreadfully medical emergencies could spin out of control at hospitals came early in his life when, as a young resident, he watched with horror a mass of critically injured patients surging into the emergency room of his hospital, crying and screaming for help from the hopelessly overstretched staff. He and a team of doctors fought heroically through that dreadful night to save lives, but one after another, the seriously injured patients succumbed even as India welcomed a New Year.

In the process of recovering from the benumbing shock of that night, the young resident had grown many years older and wiser.

He realized that most people in India lived in an inherently hazardous world where such disasters were waiting to happen.

Worse still, the country's hospital system was woefully underprepared to deal with such emergencies.

Nowhere were the dangers as brutally apparent as on its roads, which continue to be among the most dangerous in the world, with an alarmingly high rate of fatalities and disabling injuries. For each death that takes place on India's roads, it is estimated that five end up suffering from permanent disabilities. The other twenty are faced with serious injuries. The country saw over 600,000 road crashes. Out of this number, 60% led to severe injuries that resulted in lifelong disability. 34% resulted in fatality. According to the World Health Organization, India has the highest number of fatal accidents globally.

Against this bleak backdrop, Dr Venkataramana's resolve grew stronger as he set about planning a system that could redefine emergency care in the country and stem the terrible tide of avoidable deaths and injuries. His plan involved adapting several groundbreaking practices he had witnessed during his training stint at the renowned Nordstadt Hospital in Hanover, Germany, and incorporating some of his own based on India's very different ground realities. The plan forming in his mind was large in scale and life-altering in scope, which, he realized, would require an organization to evolve and execute.

Dr Venkataramana is responsible for bringing together a well-knit team of dedicated individuals who come from multiple fields, including medicine. This team was able to make sure that ideas were effectively executed. Not only did they share his vision and passion, they became the backbone of his mission. This group of professionals was able to establish the Comprehensive Trauma Consortium (CTC). Such an endeavor brought a sense of structure to their goal.

Together, they worked on developing new ideas, planning strategies, and implemented them until their work showed impact.

Over time, CTC became the face of the doctor's mission. It became a melting pot of ideas, a hub for execution, and a platform for rallying support, mobilizing resources, and raising awareness among people.

It was through this consortium that his vision transformed into actionable strategies, reshaping emergency medical care in Bangalore and far beyond.

Among the most visible signs of MERSY, identified by the number 1062, were its talismanic ambulances, repurposed as mobile life-saving units. A network of outdoor first-aid clinics was established at accident-prone spots along highways and in densely populated public areas. These ambulances played a vital role in stabilizing patients during transport, thereby avoiding complications. Their timely intervention saved countless lives. In a short period, 1062 became a byword for life-saving emergency care, much as 911 is in North America and many other parts of the world.

In the connected universe of MERSY, accident sites, ambulances, police control rooms, and hospitals were all seamlessly networked, ensuring rapid and well-coordinated response to every 1062 call, mirroring 911-based systems. The doctor wanted every second after a distress call to be exclusively spent on saving lives, which in a country like India, was often best served by attending to people rather than expecting them to reach the hospital on their own. This was the logic behind the fully equipped 1062 clinics on highways and vulnerable accident spots, such as crowded bus and railway stations.

Although these plans effectively covered most bases on the ground, they left one question unanswered: how to address emergencies in distant outbacks, inaccessible by road, and far from any form of help? The obvious answer by air involved its own challenges, as the concept of air ambulances was utterly alien to India at the time. But far from being deterred by this predicament, Dr Venkataramana marched on, creating India's first air ambulance network in collaboration with the likes of Captain Gopinath of Deccan Air fame and Hindustan Aeronautics Limited. Post-take-off, this initiative not only extended the reach of emergency services but also ensured that critical care would be delivered swiftly to even the most remote areas of the country. This set a new standard for emergency medical services nationwide.

However, even the best-laid plans, backed by clear vision and committed teams, can unravel in the face of finance and resource constraints.

It was no different for a non-profit organization like CTC, except that it was fortunate to enjoy the support of several high-net-worth individuals and business leaders who believed in its mission.

Among them was Mr. Sundar Raju, the chairman of the Atria Group, who stood by CTC like a rock of support through thick and thin, contributing resources, logistics, and services across every step of the operations. Their support was what drove CTC to continue its life-saving work even in times of adversity.

Dr Venkataramana forged on in his mission. He continued to find his path through barriers that existed in the government, a lack of advancement in infrastructure, and the internalized hesitance that came from those who were resisting change due to fear.

He successfully reshaped India's emergency response system. His strong spirit and determination are the reasons behind this unimaginable feat.

Between the covers of this book unfolds an enthralling story of passion, courage, and resolve, which begins in tragedy, unfolds through several chapters of gritty perseverance, and culminates in the noblest of all human pursuits. After all, what can be more human than saving lives? More benevolent than protecting people from the dolor of a disabled future? What indeed can be more beautiful than MERSY? This testament of a doctor's victory over daunting adversities in the pursuit of his merciful mission is quintessentially a stirring human story to be remembered in the golden hour of life.

- Mr. Sridhar Raman

Chief Branding & Communication Officer, ADDS Legal AI, a DSK Legal Enterprise
Former Resident Editor, The Times of India
Editor, Special Projects Outlook Business

Prologue

December 31st, 1983

The sky was bathed in the golden hue of countless lights strung across the streets. The fragrance of fresh sweets and spiced delicacies drifted through the air, warm and comforting, like the hugs being exchanged on every corner. Laughter mingled with pleasant conversations, and greetings rang out from every direction. Friends huddling over plates of good food and drinks, swapping stories, teasing each other about the year gone by. Lovers walking hand in hand, leaning close, whispering their plans for the year ahead. Families sharing prayers and blessings, hoping for good fortune and happiness. Everywhere you turn, there is a glow; in the lights, in people's eyes, in the way they hold each other just a little tighter tonight.

It is New Year's Eve, and for a while, it felt as though every grievance had been set aside, leaving only warmth in people's hearts. On the side of Brigade Road, near an old park bench, a group of friends was ringing in the New Year like everyone else. Laughter spilling between slurred sentences, the warmth of alcohol loosening their words. Joy buzzed in the air, blending with the music, chatter, and distant crackle of fireworks. Then, another group of men arrived to celebrate at the same bench. A harmless greeting turned sour; voices rose, egos clashed. In the blink of an eye, a joyful gathering twisted into a drunken fight.

A hand reached for a glass bottle. Anger overtook reason. One rash swing, the shattering of a glass, and jagged shards drove into a man's skull. Blood began dripping onto the pavement, stark and red under the streetlights.

Panic erupted. Someone screamed for help. The friends grabbed the injured man and rushed him into a vehicle. But the celebration-choked streets were clogged with cars, horns blaring, everyone still lost in the countdown to midnight. By the time they reached the hospital, it was too late. The doctors fought for him, but the New Year had already claimed its first life.

I remember standing there, beside the bed of the young man who now lay still. His friends and family were frozen in grief, their eyes hollow, their voices breaking. In front of me was a life full of potential, wasted in a single, senseless moment.

I kept asking myself, over and over, why this happened. Where did things go wrong? Was there anything more I could have done?

It took years before the answer to these questions came to me. This book is the story of that search for answers. My journey to understand, to piece together what happened, and why, and how we could preserve life better.

CHAPTER - 1

New Year's Eve
on Brigade Road

My Residency Years at **NIMHANS**
Freshly graduated from Sri Venkateshwara Medical College, Tirupati, with a heart full of enthusiasm and passion, I joined the residency Program in neurosurgery at the premier National Institute of Mental Health and Neurosciences (NIMHANS), Bangalore. The hospital was one of the best in the country, and their Neuro center was a highly sought-after location for all types of neurological problems even four decades ago. They were equipped with all the requirements and infrastructure for providing excellent training and clinical services in Neurosurgery and Neurology. NIMHANS's postgraduate training program was also very well-established with exceptional training that equips one with clinical acumen, operative skills, and research expertise from a global perspective. The neurosurgeons trained from that institute are spread across the world with successful careers, and I hoped to be one among them.

Because of the lack of better facilities, the patient load at NIMHANS was more than we could accommodate.

People from all over the state and country will reach out to NIMHANS for proper diagnosis and treatment. Although it was said to be a referral center, many walk-in patients would come to the hospital with their concerns because of its sheer popularity.

The OPD (Outpatient Department) services, at times, used to run until 8 pm in the evening. The neuro center of the hospital was quite boutique in those days, with state-of-the-art operating rooms, post-operative critical care, a head injury unit, a stroke unit, spacious wards, dedicated pediatric neurosurgery and neurology wards, an electrophysiology unit, seminar halls, and faculty rooms. The operating rooms followed a classic British-style design, complete with a viewing gallery above. As a resident, all these facilities fascinated me. I firmly believed that with the help of such facilities, no life could be lost.

Since Neuroradiology was in a nascent stage during my residency years, we weren't just observing and studying, but we actually got to perform investigations, such as carotid angiograms, ventriculograms, pneumoencephalography, and myelograms, especially during emergencies and non-working hours. This used to provide comprehensive training to neurosurgeons, to the extent that we are still not dependent on radiologists or their reports today.

Every year, only four postgraduate students were selected on a national merit basis for this program. Therefore, I knew how big of an opportunity I had and didn't mind the hardships and work pressure. We also had memorable times due to teamwork, cooperation, and a good mentoring system from the top down.

During my residency years, Neuro emergencies used to be a nightmare. The emergency department will get loaded as the day progresses, with stroke, epilepsy, head injuries of various kinds, apart from other neurological conditions. To sort out, prioritize, and admit the most needy and critical patients with only a limited number of beds available was a daily challenge. The duty resident will report to work at 7 am in the morning and has to continue till 7 am of the next day— a 12-hour shift. Once the shift is done, we will have to report back at 8 am, after an hour of break for refreshment, to the pre-operative discussion room. All the previous day's emergencies will be discussed there, and decisions will be taken collectively with the faculty.

Then they have to get on with the day's work either in OT (Operating Theater), ICU (Intensive Care Unit), or wards. Essentially, we will be working on an average of 30 to 36 hours.

Often, by the time we reach the hostel after our duty, the food mess will be closed. However, the cook who is aware of our working pattern will keep some food aside for us. His kindness and concern have made our residency life a lot bearable. I was always a curious child, wanting to learn as much as I could. So, on non-duty days, I used to visit the library, where I would catch up on some theoretical aspects and the latest medical journals until the watchman chased me away. This may sound very difficult, but when compared to the kind of training you get, all the hardships are forgotten.

I had a wonderful training experience at NIMHANS, and those years of training eventually molded my career, personality, and skills into a successful one, establishing myself as a competent neurosurgeon.

Over the years, all the theatres and intensive care units were renovated to keep pace with advancing standards. The campus has overall expanded over the years, incorporating various sub-specialties and new departments. Though if I still take a walk around the corridors, I can picture everything as it was.

The crisis of New Year's Eve

New Year's Eve already has a track record of having a load of injuries of all varieties, more so under the influence of alcohol. This has made me often wonder whether this is the proper way to celebrate such an auspicious day. I have witnessed everything from petty quarrels to serious mob violence, and injuries ranging from simple ones to fatal ones, turning what was supposed to be a happy day into one of grief and heartbreak.

In those days, it was a big custom for people in Bangalore to gather around the Brigade Road and MG Road area. They will be colorfully decorated for the occasion, and the celebration will begin in the evening and last till way past midnight. People will go around having a lot of fun and frolic, eating and drinking, and greeting each other at midnight to welcome the new year, irrespective of their age and religion. You could taste the joy in the air.

However, once the night darkens, everything depends on the amount of alcohol consumed. Drowning in drinks and having lost their wit, people often end up creating a ruckus. There will be countless altercations, falls, and accidents around the city. That is why New Year's Eve is a nightmare for the police department. From managing the traffic and crowd to keeping the mobs in order, they will be running around the whole night. More or less, this drinking and fighting has become a tradition of sorts in Bangalore, and no New Year has ever passed without it. However, other private parties, dinners, and events among the elites will be galore all over the city.

It was one such New Year that changed my life forever. I was in my 2nd year of residency program and part of the night shift crew in the hospital. We were enjoying the quiet and exchanging pleasantries with the staff. Most of them a little sad about not being able to be with their loved ones. But once midnight struck, the hospital phones started screaming one after the other. The quiet corridor became flooded with patients and attenders. Most of them were drunk, including the ones who brought the patients in. And to our alarm, a good number of them were in highly critical condition. Everyone moved in a hurry; doctors and nurses rushed in every direction to accommodate the patients. Many required detailed investigation and emergency surgery because of the head injuries and blood clots.

What shook me to my core that day was the five deaths I had to declare. Even though I have seen patients lose their lives before under unavoidable circumstances, it was the first time for me to see so many deaths so close together that could have been avoided. It was not like the deaths where injuries were too severe, or diseases slowly beat out the medicines, or chronic illnesses that were beyond a doctor's help. These were injuries created by alcohol, carelessness, and recklessness, and could have been avoided or saved if they had been able to receive help quickly.

There was one young man who drove under the alcohol's influence and crashed his vehicle into a divider. His head injury was severe, and he had lost a lot of blood by the time they brought him into the emergency room.

We tried our best to revive him, but I had to stand there and watch as his heartbeat came to a stop. Soon after that, another patient was rolled into our operating room, his family close behind. He was celebrating with his friends in their room on the second floor, and the guy jumped out of the window, thinking it was a door. A warm gathering that turned into a tragedy. The family's cries of despair as I announced his death still ring in my ears. The third guy came in with glass shards still stuck to his head after an argument that turned into a street fight. That young man also passed away, not long after he was brought in. Similarly, two other cases were brought in. All of them are young people with so much to offer and still a full life ahead of them, and all of them died within the first eight hours, not even a day, of the new year. Throughout the night, my entire effort was put into resuscitating their lives and eventually certifying their deaths. As a resident who was fresh out of college, with still hopes for saving as many people as I can, these consecutive five deaths shook me to the core. No amount of textbooks or practical, or even the logical awareness that I cannot prevent every death, prepared me for the reality of the volatile human life. I kept asking myself how such horrible things could happen on such an auspicious day. What was the point of such reckless celebrations if one can't see the sunrise of the next day? For a moment's fun, how willing are people to endanger their entire life? The families I had seen that day will never be able to celebrate a New Year without feeling gut-wrenching pain. The grief and loss will eat them alive, making it impossible for them to forget this day.

I didn't know how to console them properly. The deaths have, for the first time, shown me the dark side of neurosurgery. How severe a head injury can be compared to other injuries. The disappointment in myself and the medical facility, and the helplessness I felt, made it impossible for me to stay there longer. Once the hectic had calmed down in the emergency room, I hand over my responsibilities to the next on-duty officer and left. I was never one for huge celebrations. Yet still, I would remember to wish my close family and friends during celebrations.

However, that day, the joy of wishing and greeting others was completely lost for me.

My mind couldn't rest, tortured by the night I had.

Next morning, as soon as it was possible, I went to meet my professor and the then director of NIMHANS, Dr. GN Narayana Reddy. I poured out my frustration and disappointment to him. Telling him about the helplessness I am feeling and the questions I have.

I wanted to know why we were not able to do much despite having the best facilities. Where did we fail? He heard me patiently and consoled me. As an experienced doctor who has been working for years, such a situation was not new to him. He could understand what I was going through. He said that it is a problem our society is facing.

He asked me to imagine the situation if NIMHANS were not there. The fate of those who sought our help last night would have been much worse, and more lives would have been lost.

He stated that Neurosurgery has many facets, and injuries that come to you are only one of them. "You should not get disappointed; rather, I would say you youngsters should find the way out of these problems." His last words turned the tables for me. Instead of brooding over how I failed, I became very pensive. It felt like my responsibility to find a solution to the problem so that nothing like this would happen in the future. With that feeling, I thanked him and went back to my duty. Though I was not myself yet.

The very next day, Prof. R. M. Varma strode into the neuro center in his trademark style—gruff-voiced, with expressive gestures, and full of his usual charm. For some unknown reason, he, too, was very fond of me. He came up to me, caught hold of my shirt, and said Why the long face? It jolted me out of my gloomy mood. Slowly, I narrated the story of New Year's night's proceedings.

He listened to my story and took me aside for a talk. He explained to me the circumstances under which he had planned and built the neuro center.

The number of hurdles they had to go through, how they had to deal with the state government and the center simultaneously, and eventually, how All India Mental Hospital got transformed into the National Institute of Mental Health and Neurosciences. I listened to him intently, fascinated by the journey. It was an effort that left a legacy.

It pulled me out of my negativity. Seeing the struggles he went through to achieve what he dreamed of gave me hope of doing the same one day. It made me feel confident in myself, thinking I would also be able to find a solution for the things that are troubling me.

Later, the developments in neuroscience were so fascinating that I became immersed in understanding brain functioning and the marvels of the unfathomable organ. My teacher, mentor, and, moreover, a cherished friend, Dr. A.S. Hegde, was a pioneer in neuroscience and helped me a lot in acquiring new knowledge. True to my luck, unbelievable developments in brain imaging technology and surgical instruments occurred in the coming years. Operating microscopes transformed neurosurgery into micro-neurosurgery, adding a new level of sophistication, safety, and the demand for refined skills, along with a quiet sense of pride in the craft. Over the next three years, I immersed myself in mastering these techniques, while the management of head injuries, once central to my work, slowly moved to the background.

Soon after my residency, and after acquiring an MCh degree (Magister Chirurgiae, which means Master of Surgery in Latin), I was appointed as a faculty member and became an Assistant Professor, delivering clinical, academic, teaching, and research activities. Continuing my journey within the same institution, from a trainee to faculty, brought with it many advantages. Beyond the comfort of familiarity and a deep sense of belonging, it allowed me to grow quickly, advancing at a pace that might have taken much longer elsewhere.

Around that time, I had the opportunity to set up a neurosurgery department at a newly established, one-of-a-kind private hospital on the old airport road. I embraced the challenge without hesitation.

Back then, neurosurgery had yet to find its footing in private practice, its meticulous and demanding nature often discouraging such ventures.

Even so, the Manipal Institute of Neurological Disorders (MIND) soon earned its place as a credible, premium center for neurological care in Bangalore's private healthcare landscape.

Despite my career growth, I was still very immersed in honing my operative skills. Advances in newly introduced microsurgery skills demanded further training. That was why I decided to gain more exposure by working in foreign countries. I wanted to learn their treatment methods and newly developed techniques, which in those days were only available in developed countries.

Micro neurosurgery training in Germany

My first destination was Hannover, Germany, to work under Prof. Masjid Samii, a well-known Micro neurosurgeon and a surgeon par excellence. I worked at the Nordtstud hospital, which has a beautiful setup for neurosurgery. Prof. Samii was internationally renowned for his work in acoustic neuroma surgery, especially for preserving the facial nerve and even achieving hearing preservation—feats that seemed almost impossible at the time. Watching his meticulous handling of the brain and its delicate nerves opened my eyes to an entirely new technological perspective.

That center was already ahead of its time, pioneering microsurgery and introducing techniques and technologies I had only read about before.

Beyond the surgical skills, I learned something equally valuable: an organized way of functioning, a disciplined work culture, professional etiquette, an uncompromising commitment to quality, and the importance of punctuality.

In the basement, a fully equipped research lab gave every student hands-on exposure to research methodology, making learning a complete experience. Looking back, that program didn't just sharpen my skills—it transformed my perspective.

The Value of Time

One day, I was in the emergency department, casually observing and interacting with German colleagues to learn how they handled emergencies. While we were chatting with the duty neurosurgeons, a call came from the police department about an accident that had occurred far away on a highway. The police gave such a clear description of the scene and the injured, and there were no questions left to ask from our side. They also informed of the possibility of a significant head injury, as he was unconscious and needed to be extricated from the car. The police accomplished all that efficiently and successfully. By the time they got the patient out of the car wreck, a fully equipped ambulance came to the site. The crew examined him, took charge of the situation, and loaded him into the ambulance.

From then on, all information about the patient's vital signs, status, first aid, and support provided, including intravenous fluid administration and airway status, was reported to the hospital seamlessly. Even the arrival times were notified beforehand so that we could prepare to receive the patient. By the time the ambulance pulled up at the emergency department, all the required teams were summoned in a coordinated fashion based on the information provided by the paramedics. Each member was suited up, following the universal precaution protocols to the letter. As soon as the patient entered the casualty, the entire team evaluated him from head to toe simultaneously. The blood samples were drawn, relevant X-rays were taken, and a quick neurological evaluation was done. In no time, he was wheeled into the scan room. The brain scan showed an extradural hematoma, so he was immediately taken to the operating room. By then, the operating room was also ready for surgery, and it proceeded from there smoothly. The clot was removed, and he was shifted to neurocritical care.

It felt like a high-stakes mission executed to perfection. Everyone knew what their job was and worked in total coordination. The interdepartmental communication was so seamless that there was no confusion or delay at any point in time.

The patient woke up with no other troubles than being surprised at finding himself surrounded by doctors.

I was simply flabbergasted by watching this scene. Even after returning to my apartment, the whole process was replaying in my mind. My old memories of that New Year's Eve resurfaced that night and made me think about the way we deal with head injuries in India.

When an accident occurs in our country, most people seem to look the other way to avoid the possible police questioning, or they will be busy capturing the moment, or they will simply watch from the sidelines.

The majority won't even think about calling for help. Even if someone called for help, it will take forever for the ambulance to arrive. At that time, ambulances didn't have any necessary equipment to do even first aid. It was simply a transport vehicle.

By the time they reach the hospital, it will have taken a pretty good amount of time, thanks to the traffic. Or worse, they would be transported in a random vehicle, with no care for the head or spinal injury. Once the patient arrives, it takes forever for the doctors and nurses to take the patient in, assess the situation of the accident, do the primary check-up, and finally take the patient in for scanning and operation. The stark contrast I felt while observing the way my German colleagues treated the patient was not in the advanced equipment (though it contributed a little)— it was the TIME.

This information was my eye-opener. We could preserve human life much better if we could efficiently transport the patient to the hospital with added support, like in Germany. Those five lives we lost on New Year's Eve could have been saved if that were the case. It made me realize how much needs to be done in India.

Another difference I noticed between the countries was in the way we valued human life. India is the second most populous nation in the world—perhaps that's why we take it for granted. In countries like Germany, where the population is not in abundance, every single life is treated with utmost seriousness. For the first time, I realized that in India, we often fail to give life the respect it deserves, simply because there are too many of us.

The third thing I observed was the commitment of the teams to do their best while on duty. Not only doctors, but also the police, paramedics, and even the ambulance drivers. They don't leave any stone unturned. They work quickly, notice every minute detail, and communicate with every concerned member efficiently.

Fourth was the efficiency with which the whole system works. Undoubtedly, the quality of services is unparalleled. My mind instinctively resisted many thoughts about how well they were organized, and gradually, I began to understand the true meaning of what it is to be a "developed country."

Until then, I had assumed it simply meant a nation that was wealthy. But I realized they are not just rich in money—they are rich in every way. Rich in resources, yes, but equally rich in thought, attitude, creativity, organizational skills, and efficiency.

That night in Germany stayed with me long after I left the hospital. Watching a life snatched from the edge of death by sheer discipline, coordination, and respect for time made me realize what our country was missing. It was no longer just about neurosurgery for me. It became about building a system where every life mattered and where no one would have to die simply because help did not arrive in time.

CHAPTER - 2

The Anatomy of Delay

After experiencing the efficient and advanced way the Germans treated their accidents and patients' lives, I was more determined than I ever was about bringing a change in India. The answer to the questions that haunted me after that New Year's Eve was finally taking shape. I was going to restructure the whole emergency response and medical care system. First, I had to start small. I decided to explore all possibilities and thoroughly understand the scenario of head injuries in the country, especially in Bangalore. The results, although not very accurate at the time due to limited facilities, were still mind-boggling. We lacked good documentation of facts or any proper systems to log data, making comprehensive studies and analysis more difficult.

At that time, by our luck, the neuroepidemiology department had just received a small grant to study head injuries in Bangalore. Led by Dr Gururaj, the project became invaluable for me. By drawing data from hospitals and police, the team created a more accurate and comprehensive picture of the situation.

Results showed Bangalore had over 12,000 documented injuries per year, excluding many minor injuries that went undocumented. Including referral injuries from other areas, the number exceeds 20,000 per year.

From the results, I analyzed the fatal injuries selectively. The data revealed that 10% of deaths occurred instantly at the scene. It is tragic but understandable. In cases of high-speed or severe impact injuries that claim lives within seconds, survival is unlikely without immediate medical intervention nearby.

What truly alarmed me was the next figure: 22% of victims died while being transported to a medical facility. This highlighted a glaring gap in pre-hospital care in India, particularly in Bangalore at the time.

Even more surprising were the remaining 68% deaths that occurred after reaching the hospital, many of them days into treatment. We may not have been a "developed" country, but I knew our hospitals were not so inadequate as to explain such a high mortality rate. These numbers challenged my assumptions. They pushed me to dig deeper, to investigate the pathophysiology, treatment protocols, and systemic flaws that could be responsible for such outcomes.

Deaths before reaching the hospital

During my investigation, several factors indicated a total lack of a pre-hospital care system or an established trauma care system. Accidents often occur in remote locations or in areas where immediate medical care is unavailable. There will be no facility for any kind of help in the near vicinity. Only bystanders who may help victims if they are considerate. Most of the time, what happens is them walking away or driving by, in fear of police interactions and related legal issues. Even if they come forward to help, there will be a challenge in getting an ambulance for the victim's transportation. Most of them don't know what number to dial, and even if they manage to contact an ambulance, the drivers may take time to reach the accident location, or even worse, arrive late due to inefficiency.

I remember the time when I was about to exit the Bangalore airport after a trip, and saw a commotion happening. When I looked to see what had happened, I saw that a person had collapsed. By that time, I was almost out of the airport and couldn't go back inside. I left the airport and was wondering what to do when I saw an ambulance outside the gate. I quickly went there and informed the driver that there was a medical emergency inside the airport, and that he should proceed as soon as possible. The driver was standing outside the vehicle chatting with someone. He listened to me and said that he would go inside. With relief, I went back to my taxi.

But even by the time I loaded my luggage, the ambulance driver was still chatting and didn't appear to have any plan to get back in the vehicle and save that man's life. It was a shock to see someone taking their time to save a life in such a careless manner. I had to go back and make sure that he took the ambulance inside the airport. I stayed until the patient was loaded into the vehicle before continuing my journey.

Even if an ambulance had arrived at the right time, it was simply a white van with a stretcher, offering no medical assistance or a paramedic. Only the relative or attendant will be sitting with the patient, not knowing what to do or what to look for. The associated anxiety will further prevent them from doing anything. If no ambulance is available, people turn to private vehicles. But without professional help, a panicked lift, a cramped backseat, and careless handling can end up causing more harm than the accident itself.

Even after getting the patient into an ambulance, the next hurdle is getting them to the right hospital. In a private vehicle, bystanders might not even know if there's a hospital nearby. And even with an ambulance driver, reaching one doesn't guarantee help. Sometimes there are no available beds, and the hospital turns the patient away. Other times, the facility lacks trauma care, neurosurgery, or the specialized support needed to treat such injuries.

As a result, they often end up going from one place to another before finally finding the right hospital and settling in. Then begins the lengthy process of examining the patient, evaluating the injury, and initiating treatment. By then, precious time has already passed since the moment of the accident. This is why inordinate delays are almost inevitable. Even though the city had good hospitals by then, the lack of care on the roads and during transportation continued to feed this problem.

Deaths occurring after reaching the hospital

68% of deaths, which happened *after* reaching the hospital, was a fact that shook my core. It was way more complex to comprehend and came as a total surprise.

By the time this study was conducted, the city had well-equipped hospitals with advanced infrastructure and technology. The doctors were quite competent and equally skillful.

Knowledge sharing was no longer a barrier because the internet had made it easier.

Medicines, too, were no longer scarce; even rare drugs could be sourced without much difficulty. So why, despite all this, were patients still dying in such large numbers? That question kept growing louder in my mind, day after day.

We went through the facts with care, dissecting every detail. In the end, everything came back to one crucial point: the time lost. The interval between the injury and the start of treatment, between the accident and the first resuscitation. It was where the battle was won or lost. The patient transfer system is complex and somewhat chaotic, as I have explained in the previous system. The ambulance drivers, or bystanders, have to run around to find the right place. The majority's first instinct is to go to the nearest government hospital, which is often bursting at the seams. They have to stand in long queues before getting a consultation. Consider the case of NIMHANS; as a referral hospital, everyone will likely end up there. However, many walk-in patients do as well. Without a proper system in place, assessing them and identifying serious injuries is a huge task. Add to this the recurring problem of limited beds, and many patients are simply unable to be accommodated.

In hospitals and emergency care centers, Surgical interventions are always given priority, and often non-surgical ones are referred to other hospitals. In reality, many serious head injuries may not require surgical intervention, but need intensive care. The treatment for such injuries should begin at a crucial time, but unfortunately, that time is invariably lost in the middle of all this chaos. Due to various logistical reasons, every patient who died experienced an inordinate delay in the execution of their treatment. We realized that the average gap between the time of injury and the actual onset of treatment was anywhere between 4 and 6 hours, and in some cases, even longer. That means the most crucial window is already gone. And what really happens in those crucial hours?

Primary Injury vs Secondary Injury

The mechanics of head injury tell us that there are two stages of damage. The first is known as the *primary injury*, which refers to the direct damage to tissues or organs caused by the initial force or trauma.

The damage has limited intervention options as the injury has already been sustained.

Depending on the force and severity, the brain can suffer direct damage, leading to unconsciousness, bleeding, clots, or other serious complications.

If the primary injury is the immediate impact, the *secondary injury* is what results from it. It is the subsequent damage that develops over time as a result of the body's response to the initial trauma. Often, the primary could be salvageable, but not some of the secondary complications. As the person is unconscious after the accident, they cannot take care of themselves. So, they need assistance from the very beginning. In addition, there will be signs of brain swelling, bleeding, aspiration, vomiting, fits, electrolyte disturbances, inadequate breathing, drowning in their secretions, lack of proper oxygenation, hypoxia, or shock leading to inadequate blood supply to the brain, causing significant additional and often irreversible damage to the brain. All these complications occur within the first one to two hours after the injury. Although the majority are preventable, they require proper care and a well-organized system to manage them effectively. That is why getting treatment immediately is crucial for the patient's recovery.

Finally, after detailed fact analysis, the study concluded that the leading cause of the higher number of deaths was due to inordinate delay and the serious secondary complications. If a head injury Patient comes with all these, it is impossible to pull them out as the significant brain damage has already been established. Despite having good hospitals and experts, many efforts end up futile because of the delay and the onset of secondary injuries, which account for a significant number of deaths.

Even in cases where patients do survive after desperate efforts, the story doesn't end well. The neurological recovery is poor, and the quality of life takes a severe hit.

This also explains the high number of lifetime disability among survivors, showing a direct correlation with the timing of treatment. For every single death, five others are left with lifelong disabilities.

In 2000, the number of reported accidents was approximately 8,000 to 9,000. Out of these, nearly half were caused by road traffic accidents. In fact, 50% of all emergency hospital admissions were injury-related.

Among them, about 15% did not survive, adding up to an average of 800 to 1,000 deaths every year. To put it in perspective, on average, an accident was happening every six minutes. The data also showed that more than 140000 injuries were reported in the country. What made this even more striking was the age group of the injured, 15 to 45 years, the most productive years of life. Most of them were the breadwinners of their families. So, beyond the obvious toll of death and disability, the impact carried a heavy social and economic cost. And yet, these losses were never formally accounted for, either by the city or by the country.

Around that time, we had another set of statistics that showed India had 4 million vehicles, resulting in 90,000 accident-related deaths, whereas developed countries had 140 million vehicles, reporting only 39,000 deaths. The deaths per 1000 vehicles were 2 /1000 in the USA in comparison to 140/1000 in India. This was quite alarming. Several factors may contribute to these numbers, including poor road conditions, inadequate vehicle maintenance, reckless driving practices, a flawed licensing system, and insufficient vigilance.

Another striking detail from the study was the breakdown of causes behind these deaths. Road accidents alone accounted for 50.1%. Assaults came next, at 27%. Falls from heights or objects accounted for approximately 10%, while the remainder were attributed to various other forms of violence and miscellaneous causes. Among the injuries, direct head injuries contributed to 33%, craniofacial injuries 37 .5 %, spinal injury 3%, upper limb fractures 30.2%, and lower limb fractures 37.7%. One can notice that the majority of the injuries had an impact on the head, directly or indirectly. Major cities like Bangalore have a large number of two-wheelers, but the enforcement of safety gadgets is very careless.

Helmets were left to people's choice, and seatbelts were not a standard design in most cars. The overall scenario of traffic safety was quite pathetic. However, this analysis provided us with ample scope for introspection.

Introspection

The available data provided me with a lot of information, insight, and a variety of ideas that will help me create a viable system. I decided to pinpoint the causes that are primarily responsible for such a high number of deaths. Only then could we think of addressing them in any meaningful way. Of course, I was aware of the sheer scale of the challenge. Too many problems, too many stakeholders, and too many systems deeply rooted in traditions. None of this could be changed overnight.

So, I decided to treat the problem as a single entity, with one single, clear goal of reducing death and disability. I worked backward, step by step, using reverse analysis to uncover the real obstacles. After months of thinking, rethinking, and validating, the picture became clearer. The key problems responsible for these preventable deaths were;

1. Poor access.
2. Lack of a communication system.
3. Lack of organized and safe transportation.
4. Inordinate delay.

Of the four, most pointed toward issues outside the hospital. Yet, when seen as a whole, the results gave a misleading picture as if the real problem lay within hospital care. However, that wasn't the case. Hospital care was already dynamic, constantly evolving with the new technologies and improved practices. So, instead of chasing that, I chose to begin with the challenges that were outside the hospital.

I was also able to reach a few definite and convincing conclusions that support the idea that head injuries and accidents are preventable. Even if the primary injury cannot be avoided, taking the right efforts can prevent the secondary complications that usually arise due to delays in treatment. Therefore, the future steps had to align with the *timeline*. Without that, all the expertise and effort that specialists put in would continue to go to waste. With this evidence in hand, I began shaping the model.

1. Poor access - India has never had an emergency helpline number like those in other developed countries. In an emergency, no one knew which number to dial, and they ended up transporting the patient in private vehicles without proper assistance. For people in rural areas, even that was not possible. The only accessible number anyone knew was 100, the police control room. However, the police jeeps are meant for crime management and vigilance, not for medical emergencies. They had no stretchers, no medical kits, and no trained personnel on site. Unlike in the US, where 911 had been in use since the late 1960s, or in Europe, where 112 was standardized across countries, India had no single point of contact for emergencies. Each state has its own numbers for ambulance, fire, and police, but very few people knew them, and even fewer had phones at home to call from at that time. In rural areas, the situation was even worse. Poor telecom infrastructure meant that help was often out of reach altogether. Those who could get through often found that there was no centralized coordination between the police, ambulance services, and hospitals. As a result, many patients were rushed to hospitals in autorickshaws, private jeeps, or even bullock carts. Even if they happen to get an ambulance, there is still no connected system to guide them to a hospital with available beds or facilities. The helplessness of bystanders and families was palpable; panic, confusion, and delays ensured that the "Golden Hour" was lost. The lack of coordination between the various components of the emergency medical system proved to be one of the greatest obstacles in saving lives.

2. Lack of a communication system - Communication was poor, and mobile phones were not available at the time. So in an emergency, people had to rely on public telephone booths. Imagine the panic of trying to find a working booth, standing in line, or dealing with a broken connection while someone's life was hanging by a thread.

Even if you somehow manage to connect with a hospital, most of the time, the receptionists won't show any sense of urgency and will keep the phone on hold or take their time in sending an ambulance. It was an utterly futile system to depend on when every second mattered.

3. Lack of an organized or safe transport system - First off, we had no proper concept of an ambulance system. The few that existed were in poor condition and tied to their respective hospitals, with no centralized service or organized medical transport.

An ambulance was nothing more than a white van with a stretcher inside, sometimes accompanied by the bare minimum of an oxygen cylinder, if one was lucky. There was no paramedic system, no trained staff to provide life-saving care en route, and certainly no protocols to handle emergencies on the move. Unlike in developed nations, our ambulances had no privileges and no right of way on the roads, no special lanes, and not even public awareness about moving aside to let them pass. Even the police were largely ignorant of such needs. On top of this, the chaos of traffic in growing cities made the situation worse. The blaring sirens meant little; an ambulance would be stuck in the same congestion as everyone else, often forced to crawl through the streets while the patient's precious minutes slipped away.

4. Inordinate delay - All these factors, whether independently or collectively, contributed to the unacceptable delays. People, out of ignorance and helplessness, ended up becoming obediently accommodating to the system. Everything else was surrendered to fate and destiny, as though nothing could be changed.

Unavoidable Truths About Accidents and Head Injuries

- Accidents are unpredictable—they can strike anyone, anywhere, at any time, and are a major local hazard with global significance

- Accident-related deaths and disabilities are largely preventable, but the existing systems and infrastructure are inadequate to meet the growing demand.

- With better coordination of existing resources, outcomes can improve significantly, even without massive new investments.

- Immediate, synchronized, streamlined trauma care can save lives.

- Among all injuries, brain trauma is often the leading cause of death and long-term disability.

- The brain is an extremely sensitive organ; even a few minutes without oxygen, blood, or glucose can result in irreversible and permanent damage. Unlike other organs, damaged brain tissue cannot be repaired or replaced.

> - There is an urgent need for advocacy, public awareness, and system-level intervention to address these preventable tragedies.
> - Time is a critical and decisive factor in saving lives and preventing permanent damage.

Golden Hour

After identifying the reasons for the high number of deaths, the next big question was *how* to go about it. These issues regarding the death numbers were not something that could be solved overnight or with a single idea. The thought process continued relentlessly for months, involving repeated thinking, rethinking, and weighing of possibilities. Slowly, a tentative plan began to take shape. The focus was clear: if we were to make any real difference, we had to first tackle the three cardinal issues of access, communication, and transportation.

I had confidence in the capability of our hospitals and the expertise of the doctors once the patient was inside. That was never the real problem. The real challenge lay outside, on the roads, where precious time was slipping away. Therefore, the utmost priority was to reduce this time lapse. This is where the concept of the Golden Hour took center stage. I began vehemently promoting the idea and its undeniable benefits. The Golden Hour refers to the first hour immediately following a traumatic injury.

Medical science has repeatedly shown that this single hour is the most decisive period for survival and recovery.

If a patient receives proper care within this window and gets their airway secured, bleeding controlled, and vital functions stabilized, the chances of survival increase dramatically, and the likelihood of long-term disability decreases. Once this window is lost, even the best hospitals and most skilled specialists can only do so much because irreversible damage may already have set in. The Golden Hour, therefore, was a mission for me. Not a medical concept. It was a rallying point. I wanted everyone, including policymakers, doctors, ambulance staff, and even ordinary people, to understand that saving a life begins before the hospital, and every single minute counts.

Comprehensive Trauma Consortium

To achieve this, I knew I had to design a decentralized model that could coordinate and synchronize with the numerous existing resources we have. Building a completely new system from scratch was neither practical nor sustainable. The best option available to us was to take what we already had, reorganize it, and make it function more

efficiently. Out of this idea, a non-profit NGO, the Comprehensive Trauma Consortium, also known as CTC, was created. Each letter in its name carried meaning and responsibility. The first "C" stood for *Communication*, because without timely information and coordination, nothing else could move forward.

The "T" represented *Transportation*, the backbone of emergency response, ensuring that patients reached the right place at the right time. The final "C" stood for *Care on the Road*, because survival often depended not only on reaching the hospital, but also on what happened during those critical minutes in transit. It was not just a name, but a commitment and a structured way of saying, We are here to fix what has been broken for far too long. Establishing and synchronizing all these elements was the next major task. It required reaching out to numerous individuals, including officials, government agencies, the police, and anyone who could offer insight or support. Countless discussions were held to shape this initiative into a credible and functional entity. During this process, my close friend, Mr. C. Venkatesulu, a chartered accountant, suggested that the best course of action would be to form a trust and register it as a non-profit organization. His suggestion became the turning point. Not only did he guide me through the entire process of establishing and registering the trust, but he also continued to serve as one of its trustees.

Many people in the medical field were excited about this idea, like Dr. Sharan Srinivasan, then a young and dynamic neurosurgeon who played a very active role in the initial stages. Later, Mr. A. Jagadish and Mr. Gururaj Rao came forward, extending unwavering support to every activity we undertook. Also, Miss. Vijayalakshmi and Miss A. Vijayalakshmi provided huge support in maintaining all the admin operation at the CTC from the very beginning. However, I had also faced rejections and harsh criticisms from many sides when I pursued this idea. Especially from government hospitals, which believed that what I was doing was undermining their work and was criticizing them. It was never the point. All I wanted was to improve the pre-hospital care, which many failed to understand. Their resistance was certainly disheartening. This is why, during the initial years, we primarily worked with private hospitals.

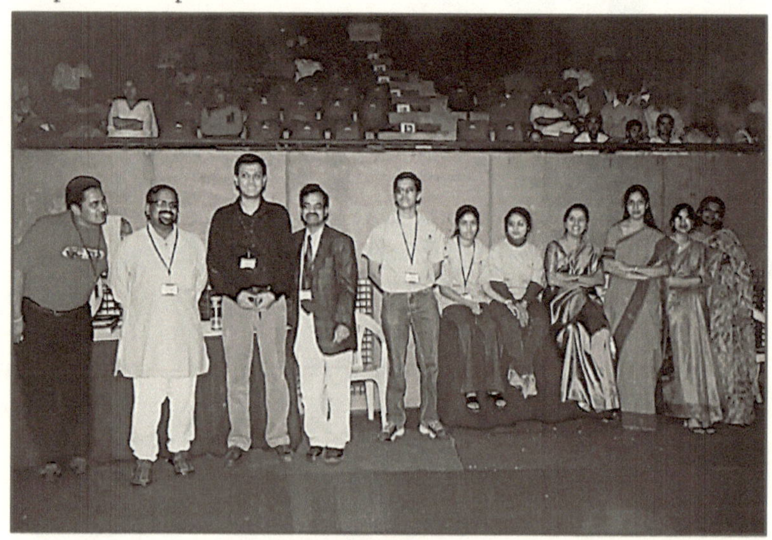

CTC Team

Over the years, the idea began to take root in many hearts, and more and more people joined me on this journey. I recall the numerous meetings I held at my home with colleagues and partners, as well as the ones that took place in the commissioner's office and small restaurants, where we would sit together for hours, brainstorming, debating, and refining our ideas. We planned, we executed, we learned from our mistakes, and we kept evolving. That rhythm of constant learning, unlearning, and improving was what truly shaped our success. Once CTC was underway, our attention naturally turned to the next big challenge: communication.

CHAPTER - 3

Dial 1062 : India's first trauma hotline

A quiet evening. You are enjoying a night drive through the outskirts of the city. As you take a turn, you stumble across an accident site. A car has crashed into a tree, and three passengers inside are hurt. What will you do? You alone can't move the injured passengers into your vehicle, nor is it advisable to do so, as it can worsen their injuries. The next logical step is to call an ambulance. But here's the question: *which number will you dial?*

One thing that fascinated me during my visits to developed countries, such as the USA and Canada, was the simplicity of their emergency response systems. They have a single emergency number, 911. Whether you need the police, fire department, or an ambulance, that one number is all you need to remember. The call immediately connects you to an emergency dispatch officer, who then contacts the required service and dispatches them directly to your location.

Their technologies are so advanced that the very moment a distress call is made, the caller's location automatically flashes on the dispatch system, enabling responders to reach the spot without delay. That is not the case in our country. Take the case of Bangalore, for example; each hospital has a unique number for its ambulance service, which the public may be unaware of. Even the government-established numbers like 100 and 102 were not widely known, and very few citizens were actually aware of them. So, in the face of an emergency, people would often scramble in confusion.

At least today, with the help of the internet, you can quickly locate the nearest hospital or ambulance service.

But back in those days, when we first began this mission, things were far more complex and uncertain.

What we needed was a control room of our own to manage and coordinate all the calls, as well as a designated number for emergencies. We began by using the police department's emergency helpline, as it seemed to be the most reliable option at the time. After all, in moments of crisis, people often turn to the police for help. Although the number was few due to the stereotype of police being scary.

We worked very closely with Mr. Ajay Kumar Singh, the Additional Commissioner of Police, and Mr. M. N. Reddi. Every Saturday afternoon, we would meet at Sri MN Reddi's office to discuss logistics. Initially, a dedicated station was given in the police control room itself. The first control room was set up at Infantry Road, and the people in there were quite cooperative. All the calls were landing on the number 100, and they were well received, but the operation was nowhere near running smoothly, as it had too many side branches.

The first challenge was to filter out genuine medical emergency calls from the numerous other requests flooding the police helpline. There was also the issue of certain calls not being meant for a non-police person. Therefore, it was challenging to navigate all these rules and regulations. Once we filter out the medical emergency calls, all the necessary details, such as the location and state of injury, must be noted. After that, we will need to locate the closest ambulance, communicate with them, and provide all the necessary details, then dispatch them as quickly as possible. Once the ambulance arrived at the accident site, the next step was to safely transfer the patient to the hospital. We will notify the nearest hospital to ensure that a bed and medical team will be ready upon arrival. This required continuous tracking and coordination until the patient was handed over. However, in practice, the logistics often broke down—there were communication gaps, a lack of ambulances on time, delays due to traffic, or a lack of preparedness at the hospital side, which all jeopardized the entire effort.

Over time, these cracks in the system became impossible to ignore, compelling us to seek stronger and more reliable solutions.

In those years, mobile phones were still a luxury for the majority of the population. Even in the bigger cities, landlines remained the primary means of communication. Paging technology had only just begun to emerge, and BSNL landlines were the most dependable, and often the only, means for people to stay connected.

Our idea was to secure a fancy, easily memorable landline number for CTC. For this, I visited the BSNL zonal office in Ulsoor. The officials there were supportive, and without hesitation, they allotted us a number. Around the same time, we also became aware of the concept of toll-free systems and abbreviated numbers, which could make access even easier, and we began actively propagating them. It was during this time that the then Indian Minister of Telecom, Mr. Dayanidhi Maran, visited Bangalore. Knowing he was staying at Leela Palace, we decided to meet him at 8 p.m. He was young, dynamic, and a remarkably receptive person. What struck me the most about him was how patiently he listened to what we had to say. He assured us of his support and asked us to meet him again in Delhi to take the matter further. When we went to Delhi for an appointment, he was kind enough to remember us and immediately signed our application and directed us to an IAS officer. Even after this meeting, we continued to communicate for a while.

During our second visit, we met an officer from Guntur who assisted us in processing our application. I spoke with him in Telugu and explained the concept to him. He took the time to review our paperwork and promised to do his best efforts. Within a few months, BSNL allocated Number 1062 to the Comprehensive Trauma Consortium. Not only did we consider it a huge achievement, but we also treated it as a defining milestone in our journey.

However, we didn't get a moment to relax. The next set of logistical problems hit us again. We thought that once the number is allocated, it would be easy to install. However, the number first needs to be approved by the local BSNL office. We also needed to create a line on which these calls will land. Given the complexity of the issue, my friend at BSNL, Mr. Naidu, offered to help us. Mr. Naidu and his colleague, Mr. Someswara, handled all the logistics-related issues.

At the same time, I was meeting with the authorities to obtain the appropriate sanctions. Soon, we realized that while the number would be installed through the Ulsoor exchange, it had to be individually connected to every single exchange across Bangalore to ensure citywide coverage. This process took nearly six months. Until then, calls could only be received from the local area. Finally, 1062 was established as a four-digit emergency helpline.

Dedicated Call Center

Mr. A. Jagadish, who lived in Kodihalli, was kind enough to provide an office space for CTC on the old airport road, just opposite Kemp Fort. That was a big step forward. Together, we toiled to establish a proper command center of its kind. The BSNL lines were reinstalled, and we purchased an EPABX (Electronic Private Automatic Branch Exchange) system with 10 hunting lines. The EPABX functioned like a mini telephone exchange within the office, ensuring that incoming calls were automatically routed to available lines, preventing calls from being accidentally dropped or missed. Computers were also installed, and new staff were recruited and trained to handle calls around the clock. A detailed protocol was laid down to receive, follow, track, and accomplish every emergency task with precision. The 1062 number was then connected to the system. When the display board was hung in the office for the first time, it was an exciting moment for all of us to witness. Sadly, after the new emergency number 1062 was made public, we began receiving numerous prank calls and fake calls from the public. It was challenging to navigate through all the calls and identify the genuine ones. It took some time for the public to understand that this was a genuine life-saving service, not something to be misused; however, the prank calls never completely stopped. We had to implement a system to filter out such calls, which became an additional task that consumed the next six months.

While we managed to overcome many of these initial hurdles, the misuse continued at such a scale that we were eventually forced to withdraw the toll-free access. This was a difficult but necessary decision to safeguard the service's effectiveness.

We were able to establish the call center and keep the service going only because of the support and help we received from many kind-hearted people. Mr. Jagadish, Mr. Gururaj, Mr. RT Kumar, and Mr. Paddy Menon have become active members of the center, supporting various activities. Mr. Jagdish took charge of supervising the control room. Mr. Gururaj runs a creative company called Lumos, which is quite tech-savvy, and he has created a dedicated website for CTC to handle all communications. Mr. Paddy took the initiative to build corporate connections and secure various resources. Mr. R. T. Kumar, who ran a PR agency called Oysters, extended his full support by strengthening our presence through PR and media connections.

Thus, we started progressing quite rapidly.

Communication System

Once we made a proper channel for the public to reach out for help, the second challenge lay in providing effective and seamless communication among the hospitals and ambulances. We aimed to address the issue of hospitals turning away ambulances due to a lack of available beds. This requires prior notification to the hospital, and in the event of a bed's non-availability, redirecting the ambulance to the next nearest available hospital. We explored various options, but with the systems available at the time, it was nearly impossible to create a dedicated network across the city. That's when Mr. Rajaram stepped in and offered wireless connectivity as the only practical solution. Once the decision was made, however, we were met with yet another set of logistical challenges.

We must obtain a license from the central government, procure the necessary instruments, secure a dedicated frequency allotment, and overcome the final challenge of installing towers to place the antennas. However, Mr. Rajaram did an excellent job in establishing all these. We were able to register and get the license very quickly by luck.

I personally went and appealed to the then BBMP Commissioner, Mr. Jayaraj, for permission to place our towers on utility and other tall buildings. After hearing our appeal, he gave his approval. Thus, a dedicated wireless network was established, connecting all our control rooms to the enrolled hospitals and ambulances. Throughout this process, Mr. Jayaraj communicated with me seamlessly, around the clock, and ensured that there was no interference from other systems.

Once the wireless network was established, tracking the ambulance and patient till the handover to the hospital became significantly easier. Calls were still received on BSNL landlines, but all directions, coordination, and monitoring were managed through our wireless system. This dual-channel setup proved both practical and highly effective. However, with greater efficiency came increased workload and monitoring demands. To meet this, we expanded the capacity of the control room, recruited additional staff, and appointed a dedicated manager to oversee the daily operations. Mr. Madhusudhan, our first manager, served with remarkable dedication for many years. Meanwhile, Mr. Rajaram took full responsibility for maintaining the wireless network, setting up new stations, and training the staff, ensuring the system ran smoothly.

Building a Hospital Network

The number for people to dial is set, as is the control room, and a wireless network connection. However, this is only the back-end preparation. The real crux of operations is to establish a safe medical transport system that quickly and efficiently transports the injured to the nearest hospital. To accomplish that, we first needed to establish proper connections with hospitals. Building effective communication channels was essential so that we could bring patients to the nearest suitable hospital. For this, we required data on the number of beds available, the ambulance facilities, and the medical resources each hospital could offer. With this in mind, we approached various government hospitals.

However, all government hospitals showed resentment towards adopting our idea as they were already overloaded with work.

Despite repeated explanations over multiple sessions, the concept of streamlining the system was challenging to convey. The hospitals strongly insisted that they were already doing their best and ended the discussions there, which was quite disappointing for us.

Eventually, we realized that limiting ourselves to government hospitals wouldn't take us far, so we decided to include private and corporate hospitals as well. This meant we had to modify our model. Ultimately, it enhanced the system's effectiveness and also provided us with the opportunity to expand and cover the entire city.

We turned our sights to every possible hospital. As part of the enrolment process, we collected data on facilities available in the hospital, including the availability of emergency services, diagnostic facilities, trauma services, the number of beds, and ambulance services. Though it was tedious, it eventually helped us in choosing the right options. After thoroughly evaluating the data, we approached the authorities of all the selected hospitals individually. Some agreed and consented immediately, while others took their time, and some required perseverance.

However, with all the effort, only 7 hospitals signed up before the inauguration and launch. However, over the next two years, with continued effort, the number grew to 45. The hospitals that enrolled were asked to provide a dedicated ambulance for this service and share regular updates on bed availability. We also installed a wireless system in each of these hospitals to ensure dedicated communication. This way, the wireless network extended to both hospitals and their ambulances, operating on a single-frequency system.

Official Launch on March 18, 2000.

With all the preparations in place, we were all set to launch the program and dedicate it to the city of Bangalore. We first approached the city police commissioner, Sri T. Madiyal, and other notable figures, Dr. Ajay Kumar Singh, and M. N. Reddi, who assured us of their support. After that, we reached out to Sri S. M. Krishna, the then Chief Minister, to inaugurate the program.

We received a launch date from the CM's office, and the event was planned at St. Joseph's School auditorium, located next to Mallya Hospital. Being a central location, it was a convenient choice for everyone.

Two days before the official launch, we organized a press meet at Hotel Atria to ensure that the public was aware of the program. Mr. Sunder Raju generously provided all the facilities at the hotel, including high tea, to all the personnel present, that too completely free of cost. Mr. R. T. Kumar managed all the logistics for handling both print and electronic media, while Mr. Ajaykumar Singh represented the Police Department. The meeting went smoothly, and the media responded positively to the new concept and initiative.

After the press meet, we got busy with stage arrangements at the main venue. The launch was scheduled for 9:30 a.m. on March 18, 2000, and we were all set for the new beginning. However, in the evening before the 18th, we received a call from the CM's office stating that he can't attend, as Smt. Sonia Gandhi is coming to Bangalore on short notice. The chief minister is supposed to receive her at the airport, and unfortunately, our event was removed from the program. Since we have not made any alternative arrangements, we decided to meet with the CM and request it personally in the hope that he will change his mind. We went to his office and waited. At 8 pm, we were able to meet him and request his presence. He was quite considerate after listening to our story and gave us an alternative that would work for him. He cannot cancel going to the airport since it is a protocol, but if we can reschedule it to 8 am, on the way to the airport, he will stop by and do the honors. We were thrilled with that option and assured him that we would have everything ready by 8:00 a.m. the next day.

Soon after leaving the CM's office, we started making all the necessary arrangements. We called all the guests personally and informed them about the changed time. We had to work till midnight to rearrange everything. On the day of the inauguration, all the Ambulances were brought and parked for the launch in the early morning itself.

On the dais, Prof. R.M. Varma and other dignitaries were seated, and the Chief Minister came exactly at 8 am. He was really surprised after seeing all the arrangements we made and the number of people gathered to witness this moment.

He decided to spend more time with us after seeing the crowd. There was a brief, formal welcome, and I presented the concept to everyone. Later, the project was officially launched and dedicated to the city of Bangalore by the CM. He addressed the audience and was in no hurry to leave. The inauguration went well beyond our expectations. He later came out and flagged the ambulances. Finally, he arrived at the wireless station we had set up and formally inaugurated it. He even connected to a hospital through the wireless network before leaving for the airport. After that, everyone gathered for a light breakfast.

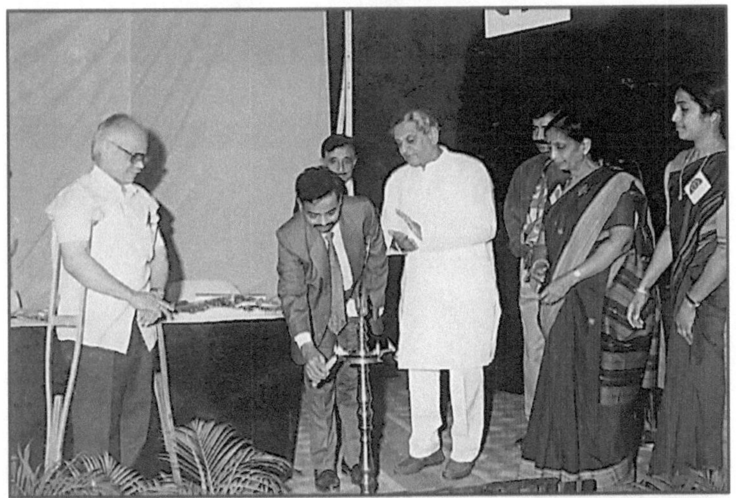

Inauguration of CTC by Chief Minister S. M Krishna

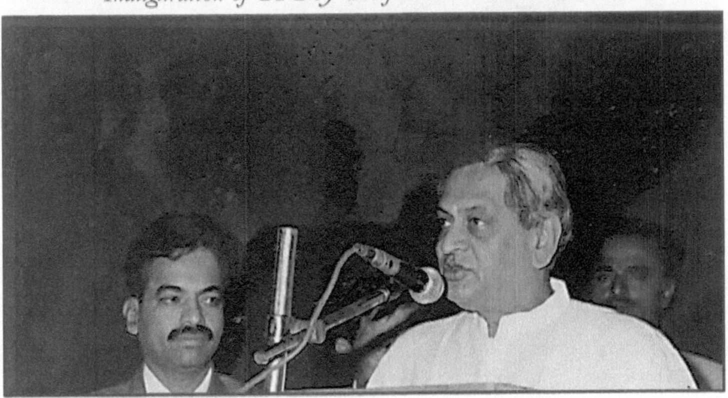

Address by Chief Minister - Sri S. M Krishna

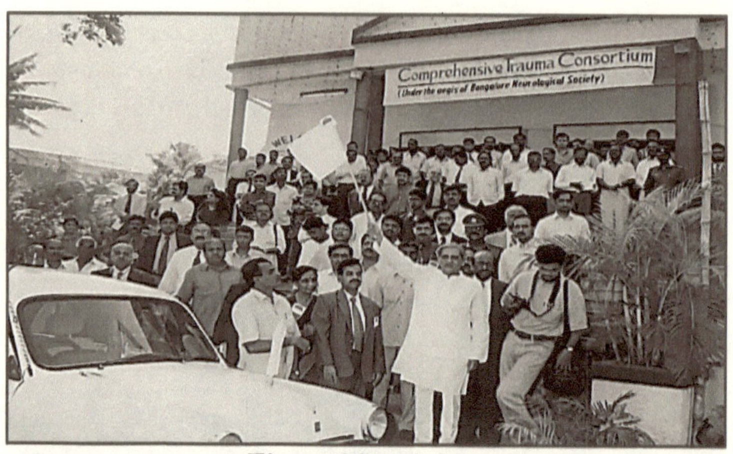

Flagging Off Ambulances

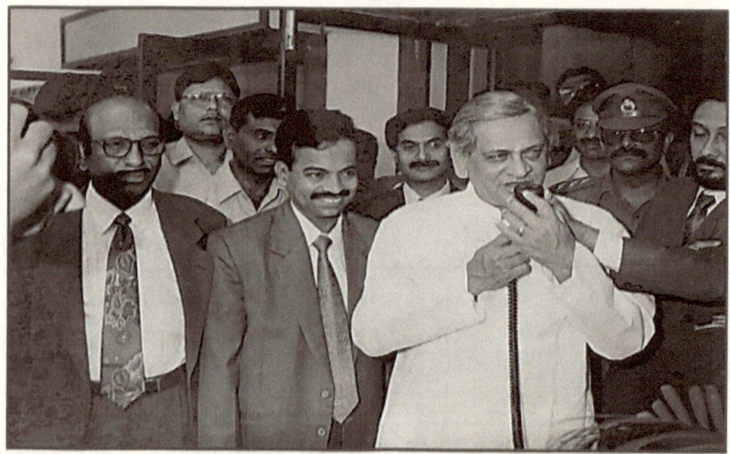

Inauguration of Wireless

The event received good media coverage, and awareness started to grow. This helped us reach out to more hospitals and encourage their participation. Our entire team then plunged into action, working on multiple fronts to move the initiative forward.

For the first time, Bangalore had a dedicated trauma hotline, 1062, and a system that gave people a number to call. It was not just a launch but the proof that with persistence, collaboration, and belief, even the most impossible ideas could take shape. As the sirens of those newly flagged ambulances echoed through the city, I knew this was only the beginning of a much larger journey.

CHAPTER – 4

From White Vans to Mobile ICUs

ASafe Medical Transport System
After the launch, our entire focus shifted to providing quality service to those in need. Since it was a new concept, we were rolling out the plans and simultaneously learning from them as they were being executed. We continually worked on our rules and regulations, refining them as the situation demanded. This improvisation was necessary to figure out the ideal working model. Soon, we realized that if the ambulance was located in the hospital, which had been the custom, the response time was becoming longer.

Secondly, the ambulance belongs to the hospital, although it was specifically designated for this purpose; it was also often used for other hospital transfers. Therefore, the non-availability of an ambulance at a specific time became an increasingly significant concern. Thirdly, the ambulances in those days were mere white vans with no proper equipment within. We attempted to improve the system by consulting with the hospitals repeatedly, but we were unable to reach a solution.

Hence, we restructured the model once again to address these three issues and developed a new dedicated ambulance system. First, we addressed the shortage of ambulances by appealing to every organization to donate ambulances to the cause. After a relentless effort, the first breakthrough came from Infosys. Mr. Nandan Nilekani and the then CFO, Mr. Mohan Das Pai, took a great initiative to donate the first five ambulances. This marked a significant breakthrough for the new system.

We then consulted with Tempo Travel Motors to design and create high-quality interiors for the ambulance. We needed more than just a stretcher and an oxygen tank. We provided some customized designs to Veeresh Motors that will accommodate all the necessary medical equipment inside. These designs featured additional lights, particularly a rear focus light for nighttime rescue. Additionally, ambulances require safety and visibility as they travel ahead of many vehicles to reach the hospital in a timely manner.

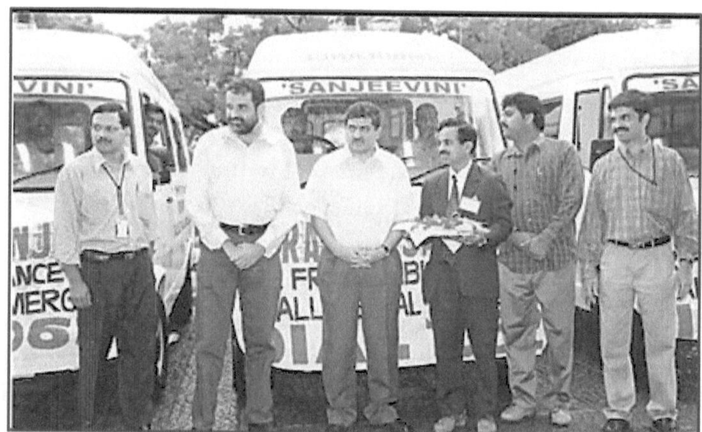

Donation of Ambulances by Infosys – Mr. Nandan Nilekhani and Mr. Mohandas Pai of Infosys Handing over the Keys

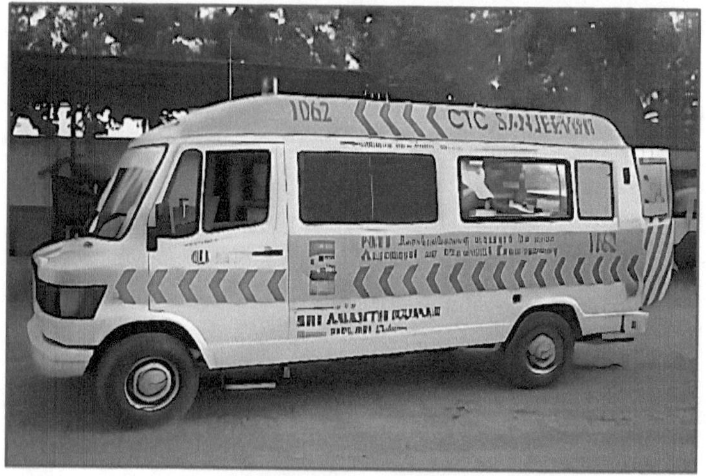

Modernised ambulance

So, from a white color, we changed the exterior to reflect a luminous color design. So that at night and in bad weather, the ambulance will be visible to other vehicles. We then established a reliable communication system in every ambulance, allowing both the control room and hospitals to reach them quickly. The patient loading stretchers were also modified to be dynamic for easy and quick use. Each ambulance was then equipped with oxygen lines and a dedicated space for a cylinder. Additional provisions were made for a suction apparatus, first aid kit, spinal board, splints, intravenous fluid setup, electronic monitors, a pulse oximeter, a BP apparatus, and a complete airway protection kit.

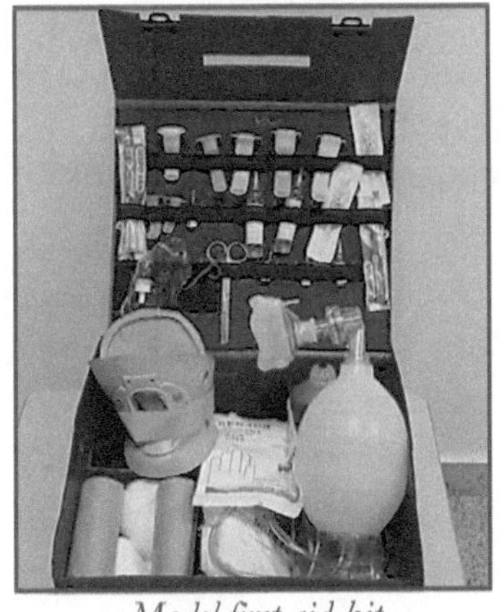

Model first aid kit

We also designed glove boxes to store adequate supplies of gloves, cotton, bandages, and other dressing materials. Emergency drugs were kept in a separate box. At that time, a German-made first aid kit cost nearly 300 DM. Since I was familiar with its design and contents, we had similar kits manufactured locally at just ₹300 each. These kits were stocked with airways, suction catheters, oxygen masks, essential medications, and dressings. They were compact and portable, making them ideal for on-site rescue.

For spine protection, we provided the design to a local carpenter, who crafted wooden spine boards for every ambulance. These boards ensured safe and quick patient transfer while immobilizing the spine. Adjustable straps were added to secure the patient during transport.

Additionally, each ambulance was stocked with cervical collars to protect the neck and Ambu bags to assist in breathing.

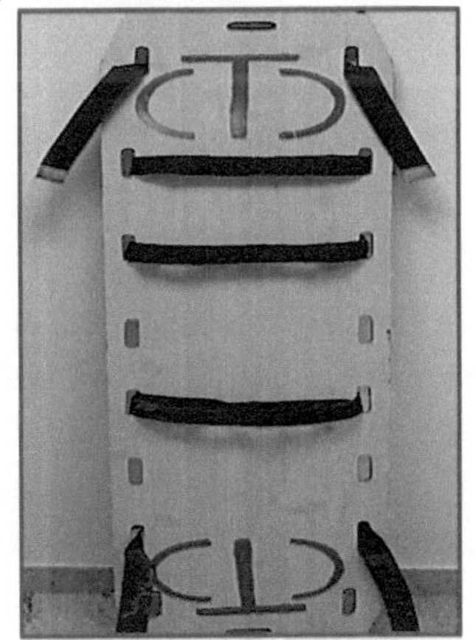

Model spine board

Later, we realized that in certain critical accidents where patients were trapped in difficult positions, the vehicle doors could sometimes get jammed. To handle such situations, we equipped the ambulances with a ladder and essential extrication tools.

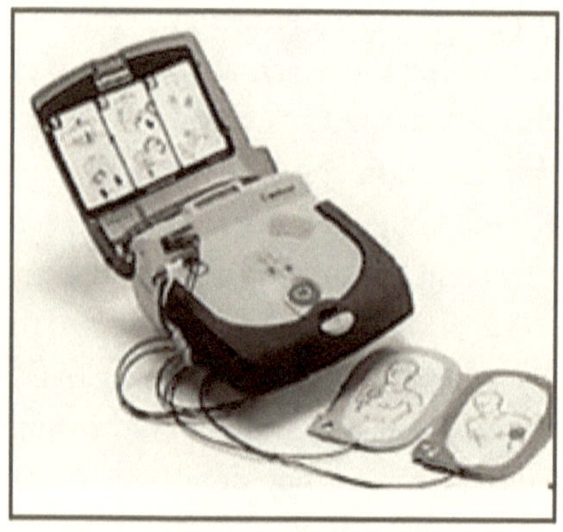

Automated external defibrillator (AED)

A year later, for the first time, AEDs were introduced into these ambulances. AED is an automated external defibrillator. The technology had just arrived in the country. It reads the patient's ECG, interprets the results, and if the heart rate is abnormal or cardiogenic shock is occurring, it can automatically administer a shock to revive heart function. Heart failures can occur during transit to the hospital, even inside the ambulance. Therefore, having life-saving equipment such as an Automated External Defibrillator (AED) on board is crucial for patient survival. Additionally, cleaning methods and sterilization processes were established to prevent cross-contamination, and the necessary cleaning materials were stored in a cabinet located inside the ambulance.

Introducing Paramedics

A paramedic is a highly trained professional who knows exactly how to handle emergency medical situations. They are skilled in using all the life-saving equipment inside the ambulance and are capable of providing critical care to stabilize patients before they reach the hospital. The concept of paramedics was not something our country was familiar with at the time. However, we realized that if we genuinely are doing all this to save lives, it is essential that we have a trained paramedic or Emergency technician in the ambulance.

We selected a few science graduates and began training them effectively. This marked the beginning of Golden Hour Academy, with Dr G. Parameswara leading the team of trainers. We were able to assign two trained individuals to each of the ambulances on 12-hour duties. The system became fairly independent,

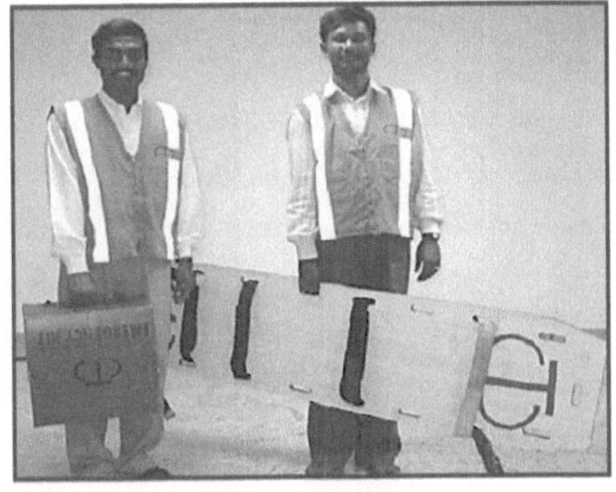

Basic paramedics

dedicated, and self-sufficient. Their services were continuously monitored. We were able to track each rescue and the performance of each individual.

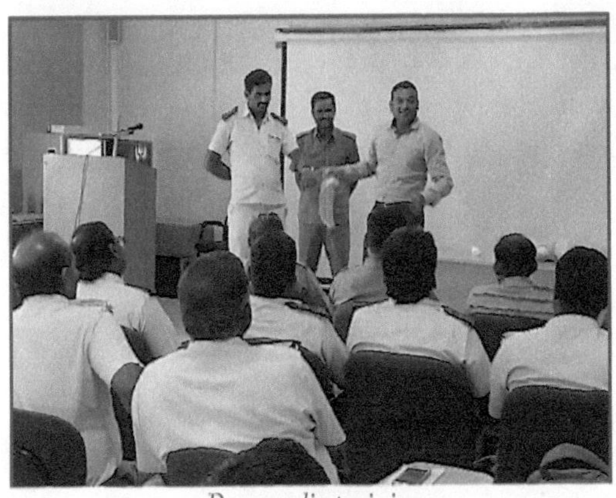

Paramedic training

Later, we decided to train the drivers as well. The idea was simple; if a paramedic was overwhelmed or an additional pair of hands was needed, the driver could step in and assist. Beyond that, we realized that learning emergency medical care would ignite a sense of responsibility and passion in them. Unlike regular commercial drivers, ambulance drivers have a unique role. They are not just drivers; they are part of the emergency response team. That is why they have to be trained in multiple aspects. First, we focused on safe driving practices, like how to prioritize cases, how to drive in adverse weather conditions, and how to navigate emergencies without compromising safety. We also trained them in professional etiquette, like understanding urgency, punctuality, and efficiency. They were taught to stay ready for odd hours, work extended shifts when required, and step in as a backup when the team was short-staffed.

In addition, drivers learned wireless communication protocols, documented basic medical facts, and followed the proper handover process to the receiving hospital, including obtaining the necessary sign-offs. All this came alongside basic medical training to help during transportation when required. For example, imagine you need to rescue a patient at night, which will be challenging due to the lack of light. To address this, we modified our ambulances by installing a powerful spotlight at the rear. When the ambulance arrives at the scene, the driver switches on this light, illuminating the area to ensure the paramedic can work efficiently and safely. The driver then steps out to assist in rescuing the patient—helping with lifting, securing, and ensuring everything is in order until the patient is safely loaded into the ambulance. Once that is done, he returns to the driver's seat and continues his duties on the road. During transit, the paramedic monitors critical vitals, such as blood pressure, oxygen levels, and bleeding points, and may initiate IV lines if necessary. Meanwhile, the driver also handles wireless communication with the control room and coordinates as required.

This teamwork ensured that patients received care promptly and effectively, even in the most challenging circumstances.

The training proved to be the right step. There were many instances where the drivers were able to act quickly and save people's lives. An incident that is still branded in my mind was when an ambulance driver and a paramedic managed to save the life of a man in a crowded railway station. The patient had suffered a heart attack while traveling in a train compartment on platform 7.

I still remember the platform number vividly. Our railway stations are not designed to allow ambulance access, so the paramedic had to grab a stretcher and run through the crowded station. They reached the platform, lifted the patient onto the stretcher, and started rushing back. Since it takes two people to carry a stretcher, there was no one left to administer care during the transfer. But in this critical moment, the driver's training made all the difference. He carried an oxygen cylinder and assisted the patient in breathing while they transported him out of the station.

Once the patient was secured in the ambulance, the driver sped to the nearest hospital, and their quick thinking and teamwork saved the man's life.

Right Time, Right Place, Right People, and Right Method

With the new ambulances, trained drivers, and paramedics in place, we focused on achieving the four 'rights.'

Right time

The fundamental goal of our mission was to perform an effective rescue and provide medical assistance within the first hour after the accident; thus, time is a critical factor. This first hour is what we call Golden Hour. Though for many other injuries we have a little larger window for rescue, unlike the fatal brain injuries, it is still important that help be available as soon as possible. To achieve this, the ambulance must reach the scene quickly, rescue the patient, and transport them to the hospital so that evaluation and treatment can begin within a critical timeframe. Ideally, the ambulance should arrive within 15 to 20 minutes after the accident. However, achieving this is not easy in our country. Our roads are narrow, lack a proper lane system, and have no dedicated priority lanes for ambulances. Add to that the chaotic driving culture, the constant crisscrossing of two-wheelers, and the absence of strict ambulance privileges, and the challenge becomes even greater. Additionally, people and other vehicle drivers often show ignorance on the road. When the ambulance is en route to pick up the patient, it must utilize all its resources to reach the patient as quickly as possible. They will use a siren even for an empty ambulance. Not knowing this, the police themselves will stop them for misusing their privilege and cause more damage. It took some time to create awareness about all these issues. Yet many things cannot be changed due to infrastructure limitations. After trying several strategies, a few essential things were implemented.

1. Relocation of Ambulance - As tradition, ambulances are parked/stationed at hospitals. We decided to place these ambulances at strategic locations instead, so they can take off from the nearest point to reach the location quickly. We sought the assistance of the police to find suitable and safe parking locations for the vehicles. Each of these vehicles will cover certain specified areas as its jurisdiction unless directed otherwise by the control room.

2. Ambulance Tracking System - Around that time, the Bangalore digital map was developed by TISL (Tata Information Systems Limited). For the first time, we had a digital map to consult while transporting the patient and tracking the ambulance's movements. TISL also had an office at the corner of Cunningham Road and was kind enough to let us use the room for our mission. We met with the authorities to incorporate these maps into the control room's computers. We conducted a couple of initial trials to assess how the system works and made modifications to suit our needs. It was customized to include information about our enrolled hospitals and their locations, as well as the locations of their ambulances. This upgradation over time helped in many ways.

Primarily, the system enables us to locate and track ambulances in real-time, thereby minimizing unnecessary movement. We can identify the nearest hospital and guide the ambulance along the shortest route. If an ambulance is stuck in traffic, we can coordinate with the police to clear the way. Additionally, we can monitor the times it takes to travel to ensure efficiency and accountability. This has made a huge difference in improving not only the efficiency of the system but also the discipline and punctuality of the drivers. The Tata Information Systems team worked closely with us and helped us reshape into an efficient version. At that time, Google Maps was not yet available in the Indian market; thus, it was fascinating to watch the entire rescue unfold on the computer screen from the control room.

3. Increasing the Fleet of Ambulances - To expand the services to larger parts of the city, the number of ambulances was insufficient. We sent appeals to every possible resource. Over time, help came from different corners. We received additional ambulances from Rotary clubs, MP Lad Fund donations, KSRTC, and several corporate donors. Even the additional hospitals that came into the system added a few vehicles. This also eventually contributed to the overall reduction in reach time.

4. Ambulance Privileges- We wanted everyone to be aware of the importance of giving way to an ambulance. First, we pushed hard with police officials to provide the right of way for ambulances. In developed countries, these norms are established and strictly followed. The moment the siren is heard, all the other vehicles should move to the left and stop till the ambulance passes. Then the traffic will resume. In addition, ambulances can stop at any place to rescue, jump the signal, and take a one-way route with safety to cut short the distance; they only need to enter with caution without causing additional accidents or problems. However, during our discussion with the police department, only a few conditions were agreed upon mutually and implemented. A direct connection was established between the CTC control room and the police control room. On a need basis, based on the emergency, we will request the police to coordinate signals and get past the ambulance. They will instruct the traffic police through their wireless network. It was a bit tedious, but it was the only viable option at the time. Police can clear the roads whenever a VIP is traveling. We took the clue from this and used it to provide the ambulance with a clear path to the hospital. We had to emphasize that VIP for us is "Very Injured Person," and a similar priority must be given to save their life. It did help in many situations to overcome the stumbling blocks. On the other hand, citizens themselves were often a major obstacle.

They try to take advantage of the situation by either blocking the ambulance or following it. However, good sense prevailed over the years, and most people now understand the importance and try to give way to the ambulance.

5. Automatic Signal Changer - After seeing our initiative and understanding its importance, some young engineering students came up with an innovative solution. They have devised a system that connects the ambulance and the traffic signal at a distance of 500 to 750 meters. A special switch will be installed in every ambulance. At a distance of 500 meters, the driver activates the switch, which in turn changes the signal to GREEN. As a result, all the vehicles in front continue to move, including the ambulance. After crossing the signal, the driver deactivates the switch and continues their journey.

In the absence of a dedicated lane for an ambulance, this seemed the best solution. We did a trial and it was very successful. We also installed a blue light that blinks while this operation is in progress to indicate the presence of an ambulance in the traffic. It worked well for 9 months. Of course, there were several obstacles in obtaining the necessary permissions, and ultimately, it remained operational only on Indiranagar, Old Airport Road, and MG Road, and gradually disappeared. We couldn't scale it up due to several logistical problems.

Nevertheless, the system became steady with time. Paramedics gained sufficient training and experience, and their confidence levels increased.

Every day, we started getting more and more resumes. To make them truly feel part of this movement, we decided to give them a new look. Mr. Sumeer Hinduja from Gokaldas provided specially designed uniforms at no cost. This has given them a very professional look and instilled a sense of pride as life savers. After sufficient training, we also gave them a badge to wear, which reads, "I am a lifesaver.".

Their morale became very strong, and they became more passionate and enthusiastic in their job. As a result of all our efforts, the results we have seen in the first two years were phenomenal. The pre-hospital death rate within Bangalore city has reduced from 22% to less than 5%. This was a great objective achievement. These figures were quite encouraging and satisfying.

We have some definite scientific evidence that the system works, produces the right results, and ratifies our thought and implementation process. It gave us the courage to make it bigger and better.

Simultaneously, CTC gained considerable popularity among both the police department and the public. The first call from the police department will be directed to our control room whenever a medical emergency occurs.

Our ambulances are also coordinated with the police department to provide coverage for medical emergencies at major city events, including New Year's celebrations at Brigade Road.

Green Corridor

All the knowledge and experience I gained while creating and running CTC eventually helped me bring new life-saving initiatives to reality, such as the Green Corridor. During my time at BGS Global Hospital, we developed a robust organ transplant program. After a patient was certified and declared brain-dead, we would coordinate with potential organ recipients and their hospitals to ensure everything proceeded smoothly. Organ donation after death requires either prior consent from the individual or permission from the next of kin. This is why we often consider patients with irrecoverable brain damage from injuries. In such cases, we would counsel families about the possibility of organ donation. If even one family agreed, nearly nine lives could be saved: two eyes, two lungs, a heart, a liver (which can often be split between two recipients), and two kidneys. This is far better than letting such precious organs go to waste through burial or cremation. Many families understood this concept. Their loved one could continue to live on by giving life to others, and they responded with incredible generosity. Unfortunately, some families firmly declined due to personal or religious beliefs, which was always disheartening to witness.

Even with the family's consent, many complications can arise during the process. I vividly remember one heart transplant during my time at the hospital. After procuring the heart, our biggest challenge was finding a suitable recipient. There was no match in our hospital or even within the city, so we reached out across the state and country to ensure the organ wouldn't go to waste. Finally, we received a call from Malar Hospital in Chennai. They had a patient with long-standing heart failure who was a perfect match. We immediately coordinated with their team and made all the necessary arrangements. Transporting an organ across state lines presents its own set of challenges, particularly because time is critical. Once an organ is removed from the donor's body, there is only a small window, based on the type of organ.

The organs are preserved by cooling them and using special preservation solutions to slow cell breakdown until transplantation. Once all the necessary clinical data and information were gathered, we instructed both hospitals to get ready.

The patient in Chennai was admitted, and all preparations for the surgery were underway.

Meanwhile, in Bangalore, before proceeding with organ harvesting, we focused on the critical steps of preserving the heart and ensuring its safe transportation. The heart must be perfused and stored in a special preservation solution at a controlled temperature, which helps maintain the heart muscle for up to six hours. To achieve this, the transportation must be completed within that time frame for the best possible outcome. For this, we required specialized cold storage systems and container boxes designed for organ transport. Everything was arranged and kept ready well in advance of the operation itself.

Then comes the challenge of transporting the organ to Chennai. We talked with traffic police and other senior police officials, explaining the concept to them and convincing them of the urgency of the situation. With their help, we identified a specific route with the shortest distance that will enable the ambulance to reach Kempegowda Airport. We ensured the road was signal-free and free from traffic. We also spoke to the airport authorities and identified the Jet Airways that corresponds to the timing of the harvest and departure. We obtained airport permissions, security clearances, and permission for the ambulance to access the tarmac and the aircraft.

The individuals who would carry the box containing the heart were identified, and tickets were booked and sent in advance for verification.

All the security formalities were completed, and they were all ready to receive the organ from the ambulance.

Once the flight timing was confirmed, we began the process of harvesting, preparing, and preserving the heart at the hospital. The heart was placed in the preservation solution and secured in the specialized container, which was then loaded into the ambulance. Meanwhile, we also assigned two trained drivers to ensure a nonstop journey, with clear instructions based on the police-approved route map. The second driver acted as a backup for any contingency. Both drivers, along with the person carrying the organ, were given proper identification tags to ensure quick security clearance at checkpoints and the airport.

The traffic police were kept constantly informed, and they effectively cleared the way to reach the airport in 40 minutes. En route, the police made several announcements to the public, requesting their cooperation and keeping them informed. It was a thoroughfare to the airport. At the Airport, the ambulance was taken through the VIP gate right up to the aircraft, escorted inside by the airport police. The aircraft was ready to take off with all passengers seated. The crew came down to the ambulance, took the box, and handed it over to the designated people who were already seated inside. Without wasting another second, the doors closed, and the aircraft departed. Air traffic control was informed beforehand to give priority to the take-off.

The plane landed in Chennai in 35minutes. Meanwhile, Similar arrangements were made at Chennai airport and with the Chennai police. The ambulance was kept ready at the designated parking bay of the aircraft. The box with people came out first and quickly left the airport. With traffic assistance, the ambulance was able to reach the Malar hospital in a very short time. The entire operation, from Bangalore to Chennai, took only one hour and fifty minutes. Meanwhile, the preparations for surgery were underway in the hospital, and the heart was transplanted successfully within the stipulated time.

The entire operation was meticulously coordinated, minute by minute, from start to finish. It took the entire day of effort with help from people across various fields, but the results were gratifying.

That day marked the beginning of the "Green Corridor" in India. This was an organized, high-priority traffic route created by the police and civic authorities to ensure that ambulances carrying organs can travel without delays, allowing life-saving organs to reach patients within the critical time window.

Inner Ring Road Menace

Meanwhile, the inner ring road of Bangalore was inaugurated. However, the road had too many crossings at multiple points, and the number of accidents spiked soon after its opening. Around the same time, KSRTC was planning an ambulance system. We collaborated with them to utilize their ambulances in a similar manner.

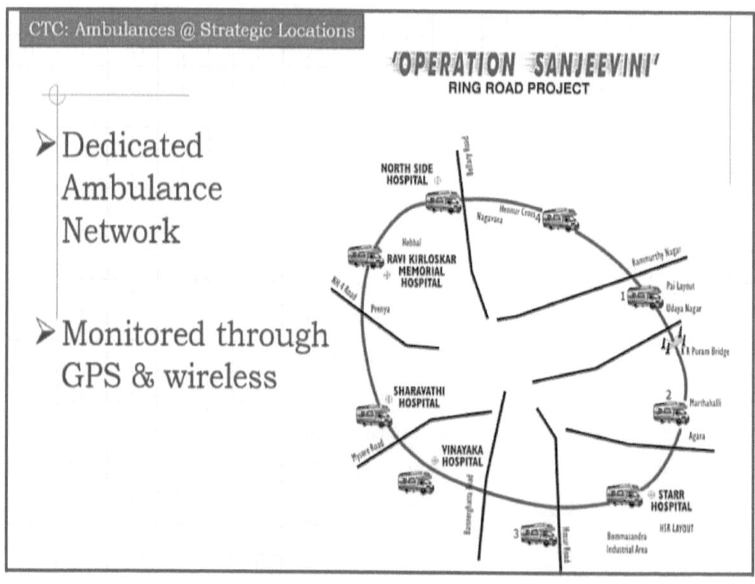

Inner Ring Road Menace

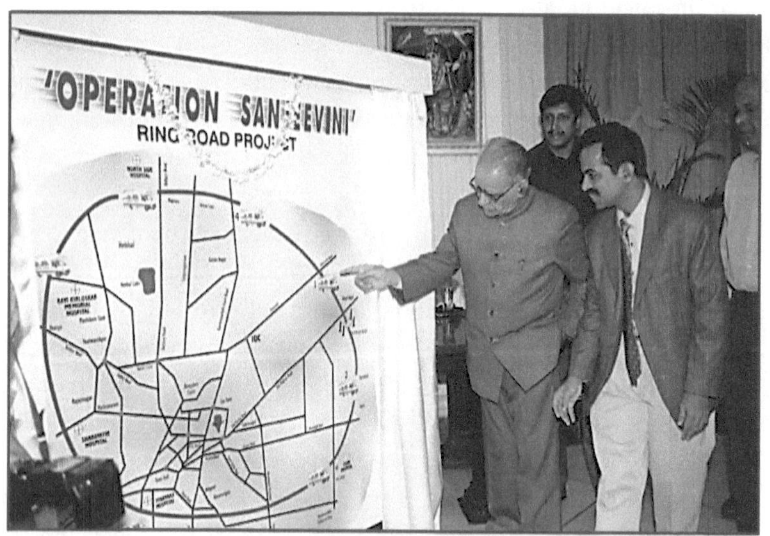

Sri TN Chaturvedi, Governor, Inaugurating Ring Road Trauma Project

For the first time, we used Swaraj Mazda vehicles as ambulances. Compared to a Tempo Traveler, these vehicles were slower and less efficient, but they served the purpose.

We strategically positioned these ambulances at key points along the inner ring road to create sector-wise coverage for the surrounding areas.

This project was named "Operation Sanjeevini" and was officially launched at Raj Bhavan by the Governor of Karnataka, Sri T. N. Chaturvedi.

The initiative proved successful, and we were able to provide timely assistance, significantly reducing deaths and disabilities resulting from accidents.

Website Launch

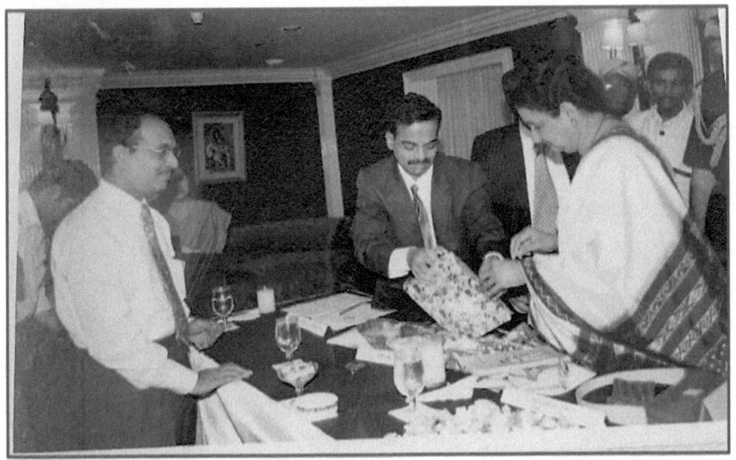

Smt Rama Devi, Governor, Inaugurating the Website

Around this time, Infosys came forward to help us build a website and dedicated a team to the task. Under the leadership of Mr. Gururaj, tremendous effort was invested in creating a state-of-the-art platform for the Comprehensive Trauma Consortium (CTC), accessible at the URL ctc.org. The website was officially launched in August at Windsor Manor by Sri Shibu Lal, one of the co-founders of Infosys, in the presence of Smt. Rama Devi, the then Governor of Karnataka.

The launch gave CTC much-needed visibility and access to various online resources. Through the website, we could make appeals, source resources, and even display daily updates on rescues. The biggest advantage was the ability to collect and maintain comprehensive data of all enrolled hospitals, including their locations, bed capacities, and other critical details, on a single system.

Air Ambulance

Most of the countries I have visited have their own air ambulance services for rapid transportation and to have quick access to remote or rural areas.

The idea was strongly appealing to me, and the confidence in establishing an emergency ambulance system and CTC led me to take a step further by establishing our own air ambulance service.

I was working at the Manipal Hospital at the time. We discussed the regulations, benefits, and challenges of establishing a helipad with Captain Gopinath, as well as the operation of an air ambulance system. The first difficulty we encountered was the lack of a suitable landing area for the helicopter. The nearest available space was in Jakkur. However, transporting the patient from Jakkur to Manipal took a lot of time, which we couldn't afford at the risk of causing the patient's death. The next solution we had was creating a rooftop helipad. Unfortunately, we didn't receive the permission for it, considering buildings at that time were not constructed with a helipad in mind. In the end, with the help of many, we successfully built a temporary helipad on the ground near Manipal Hospital.

Just ten days after inaugurating the helipad, we received a call from the US via a satellite phone. A religious leader's mother had fallen down the stairs and required immediate medical attention. She was in Penukonda, a village situated between Bangalore and Anantapur. The call was made by the devotees of the swamiji, who had a satellite phone at the time, to inquire whether we have any air ambulance service available, considering the remote location and the urgency of the situation. The call really was a surprise, considering that if it had been made eleven days ago, the answer would have been no. We discussed this matter with the hospital and Captain Gopinath. All of them were really excited about this opportunity and immediately started planning all the steps. One trouble we faced was being unable to call back, but luckily, they contacted us again, and we gave them the green flag.

We packed our first aid kit, a spine board, cervical collars, medicines, and all the necessary equipment, and sent a paramedic along in the ambulance to the airport, where the aircraft was waiting. The idea was to keep the ambulance in the airport, and once the aircraft returned with the patient, the ambulance could pick them up from the airport and bring them to the hospital. However, there was an issue regarding landing.

Because the location is a rural area with no airport or helipad, it was challenging to secure a landing space for the aircraft. We thought the aircraft would have to be landed somewhere far.

But eventually, to our relief, it was decided to land closer.

The challenge was that this wasn't a dedicated air ambulance. We had to set up everything ourselves, including permissions, oxygen masks, portable cylinders, and all the essential equipment. At that time, this was the only way available to us, so we made do. Then came the logistical hurdles. For every takeoff, we needed clearances and provisions from numerous authorities, which could take up a lot of time.

Landing was even trickier. You can't just land in a small town without preparation. We had to coordinate with local police to identify suitable grounds, arrange security, and manage the curious crowds who would inevitably gather when they saw an aircraft.

That's when I realized that we needed a proper protocol for airlifts in our region. So we developed one. After that, the process became smooth and systematic. We could quickly calculate the distance, fuel needs, identify landing spots, and coordinate local ambulances for transfers.

That first attempt taught us everything we needed to know. We transported the patient from the local ambulance to the landing ground, shifted them onto the aircraft, and secured them with all the equipment in place. It marked the beginning of a system that would later become far more organized.

Subsequently, we carried out a few more airlifts. I still remember a particular case of a patient who had met with an accident and suffered a vascular injury.

It was not a life-threatening one, but a serious limb injury where an artery was damaged. In such cases, if the blood vessel is not repaired within a few hours, the only option left is amputation. This patient was in Bellari, and we successfully managed to lift him from there and bring him in for treatment in time, saving the limb.

In total, we successfully carried out numerous cases. Each one taught us something new and added strength to the system we were building. However, we soon encountered some logistical issues that impacted the program's future.

At that time, we did not have a dedicated inventory for air ambulances. The service would often get disrupted because the same aircraft were hired by politicians during elections.

They would keep them for weeks or even months, using them for campaigning purposes. This interrupted the emergency medical service we were trying to build.

Later, we took up this matter with Captain Gopinath. After much discussion, he stated that, if dedicated funding could be arranged, he was willing to purchase a full-fledged air ambulance exclusively for medical emergencies. That was the point when the concept began to take shape seriously.

Hindustan Airlines approached us, offering their coast guard helicopter named "Chethak" for the cause. Miss Tenmozhi was in charge of modifying the helicopter to include all the necessary equipment it would need for rescue and treatment of the patient.

However, to run this operation, we needed approval from the DGCA (Director General of Civil Aviation). Sadly, because of logistical issues, we never received the approval, and we had to drop Chethak.

Over time, things evolved. The government adopted the idea, and private carriers also began to show interest. Today, air ambulances are available not only in the form of helicopters but also as fixed-wing aircraft.

Fixed-wing aircraft, of course, can only land at airports, whereas helicopters, with their ability to land vertically, can reach smaller towns and even remote locations. That flexibility made them particularly suitable for our needs.

Accreditation of Hospitals

We initiated a project to collect data on all hospitals in the city to further improve quality and care. Based on this, we developed a set of criteria and accredited hospitals accordingly, grading them based on their capacity and the range of services available, especially 24/7 emergency services.

With this system, knowing bed availability became easy even before sending a patient to a specific hospital. Daily updates from hospitals made the information accurate and reliable. We also classified hospitals into different levels and refined our dispatch protocol with clear guidelines on which types of injuries should be sent to which category of hospital.

For example, patients with polytrauma or multiple serious injuries were directed to multi-specialty hospitals equipped with critical care facilities.

This allowed the control room to play an active role in ensuring quick care by coordinating directly with hospital emergency departments. Additionally, it enabled follow-ups on patient care and outcome tracking. Over time, the data collected became more authentic and robust, significantly improving the entire emergency response system.

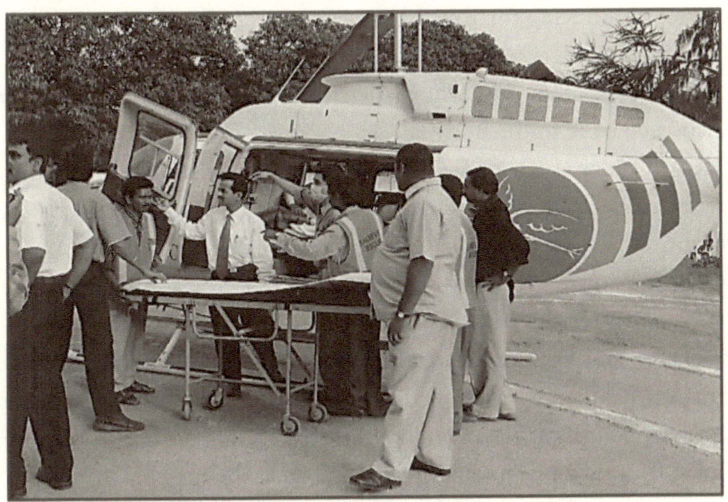

Air Ambulance Rescue on a Temporary Helipad

Decentralization

When we reviewed all the data we had collected thus far, the conclusions suggested reducing both the travel time to reach the rescue site and the return time to the hospital. That is why we wanted to introduce the concept of decentralization so that they can reach the nearest hospital as quickly as possible.

To avoid being called into two different locations and being stretched thin over large areas, we divided the city into five zones. East, West, North, South, and Central zones. Unlike the name suggests, it was not based on geography; it was based on the hospitals and their locations. We designed the city in such a way that each zone has all levels of hospitals and facilities, ensuring better reach and accessibility. Each zone was designed to include at least two Level-1 multi-specialty hospitals, several secondary hospitals, and multiple primary care centers, ensuring comprehensive coverage within the zone, except for a few special cases. The plan worked well, except for a few minor glitches. However, the patient's choice to attend any particular hospital was always respected, except in dire emergencies. This approach reduced road travel time, improved fuel efficiency for ambulances, and enabled us to consistently meet our target arrival time.

All these efforts collectively helped us achieve the objective of our mission: introducing the four right things.

Right Time – The first hour, often referred to as the *golden hour*, is crucial. During this time, the patient must be reached, rescued, and transported back to the hospital.

Right Place – The patient should be taken to the right hospital, one that is fully equipped to manage the emergency effectively and promptly.

Right People – Trained paramedics play a crucial role. They begin first aid and basic treatment the moment the patient enters the ambulance and continue care throughout the journey. Their primary focus is maintaining airway, breathing, and circulation to prevent secondary complications. Treatment doesn't stop en route; it continues seamlessly until a proper handover is made at the hospital.

During handover, the paramedics provide a complete status update, including any critical events such as vomiting, seizures, or a sudden drop in blood pressure, so that the hospital team can prioritize those issues immediately.

Right Method – Every patient is rescued following proper, standardized procedures. Unconscious patients are assessed immediately for airway patency, breathing patterns, and circulatory stability. The neck is immobilized using a cervical collar, and the patient is carefully secured onto a spine board to prevent any movement of the neck or spine.

Once the airway is secured and intravenous fluids are initiated, breathing is supported as necessary. Oxygen is administered based on pulse oximeter readings, and blood pressure is monitored periodically. Pain relief is provided, and ECG monitoring continues throughout the transfer. These steps help prevent secondary complications as much as possible. Meanwhile, prior communication with the receiving hospital ensures that the emergency room and medical team are fully prepared with the necessary equipment to act immediately. We also developed a hospital protocol to ensure that assessment and treatment occur simultaneously, thereby saving crucial time during the critical first hour.

Basic Protocol for Hospitals

In those years, emergency medicine was in its early stages and was a distinct specialty. We also decided to develop a simple document outlining all the basic and important steps to follow in each specific case of injury and medical emergency for hospitals.

We also conducted several training sessions for the staff. Later, emergency medicine underwent significant growth in the country.

At a time when emergency medicine as a course was not yet established, we took the initiative to develop a hybrid three-year curriculum in collaboration with George Washington University. As part of this program, a team of faculty members visited every two months for a seven-day session, delivering comprehensive lectures on all key topics and providing hands-on guidance in emergency departments to ensure effective clinical training.

Today, full-fledged courses in emergency medicine are officially recognized by the Medical Council of India, but this program was a pioneering effort that laid the foundation for structured emergency medicine education in the country.

Training Academy

Ambulances were an integral part of our mission. Thus, hiring trained people as ambulance crew members became an important task. If there are no trained professionals to operate the equipment, then all the advanced systems we installed serve no real purpose.

Someone must be capable of using and maintaining them effectively. From the very beginning, we aimed to create a system that could mimic or at least temporarily substitute the well-established paramedic systems seen in developed nations. Their emergency medical services are recognized as a dedicated profession.

During my international travels for neurosurgical work, I made it a point to visit and study ambulance services in every country I went to, gathering insights that could be adapted to our country's context.

The commitment the paramedics showed in the developed countries was fascinating and admirable. Their ambulances were stationed at strategic locations, ensuring the crew was always ready to respond and act swiftly. I remember one interaction I had with one of these paramedics during my visit to the fire station. The paramedic was standing outside, just taking a stroll. However, the ambulance's door was kept open. When I asked him why, he explained that the moment there is a call, he can just jump in the vehicle and move.

That was the level of training and sense of urgency they have built into their system.

Their dedication to saving lives was evident in every single action they took. This level of commitment was crucial, especially for ambulance drivers. This lack of commitment was one of the major challenges we faced in the beginning. The ambulance is parked somewhere, and the key is kept in another location, with the driver sitting in a different place or doing something else. When a call comes to the hospital, someone must first call or trace the driver.

The driver then reports to the transport head to collect keys and take instructions. Then gradually he will take a walk towards the ambulance. In the meantime, if he meets a friend, he will tell them where he is going. So much time is lost.

This system of indifference was so fixed that it was very difficult to break free from. The majority of the problems were resolved when we had dedicated ambulances and our own crew. We trained them well not only in the procedure, but also in the urgency and importance of their job, so that they became responsible gradually.

We decided to develop a system to train and educate individuals on etiquette, discipline, responsibility, and a new mindset, specifically those involved in the rescue mission.

We divided the task into various components: developing a curriculum, actual training, and creating professional courses for the future. Dr. G. Parameswara, an anesthesiologist, Dr. Radhakrishnan, a pediatric surgeon, and I formed a team to develop a simple and basic syllabus and training modules. This includes both pediatric and adult care systems.

Later, we gathered the required equipment to train. Mannequins of various types, including infant, child, and adult models, were procured. We started the basic training as soon as the training modules were ready. Simultaneously, we examined the syllabi of American, European, and Australian systems.

The original idea was to adopt one of these as such to save time. However, we realized they were all patented, and they demanded huge amounts even to use the names. So, we had to abandon that idea quickly and make our own system. Moreover, the scenarios of emergencies that occur in these developed countries differ from those in our country.

Our climate, transport systems, roads, and social situations require customized instructions. Therefore, a significant amount of indigenization was required to make the response suitable for our local situations.

Later, we rented a small space to store the equipment needed for lessons, including a projector, and created workstations for hands-on training. We then began regular training sessions. We provided the trainees with a small pocket guide containing key steps, like CPR (cardiopulmonary resuscitation), that will be crucial in saving a person's life. Gradually, more sophisticated mannequins were added, including AED trainers, as they became available on the market. All the ambulance crew members were trained repeatedly until they became adept. We wanted to expand this training program to raise awareness and educate the public.

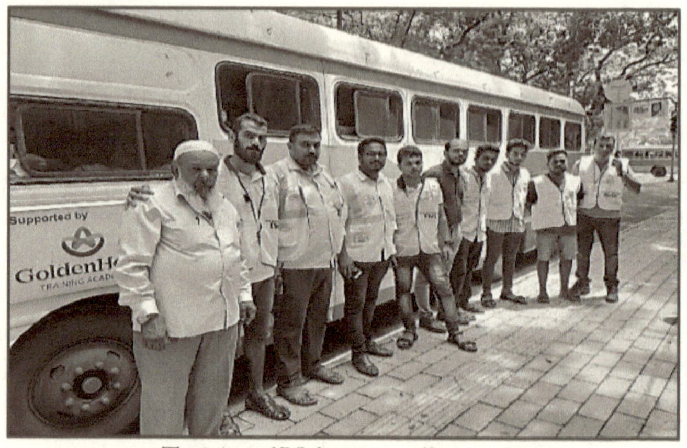

Training of Volunteers as Paramedics

The idea was simple: the more people who know basic life-saving measures, the better the chances of preventing avoidable harm. Often, common practices we do in emergency situations cause more harm than good. For example, people tend to pour water into the mouth of an unconscious person, leave them unattended on the road, or assume that they are intoxicated, all of which are dangerous misconceptions. Similarly, improper handling during transport, such as bending the neck or spine or lifting without support, can lead to severe complications. By educating people and sharing essential knowledge, we aimed to eliminate these harmful practices and promote correct, life-saving actions. The training began with police, traffic wardens, scouts, guides, and volunteers. Literally, the entire traffic police force was trained in Bangalore.

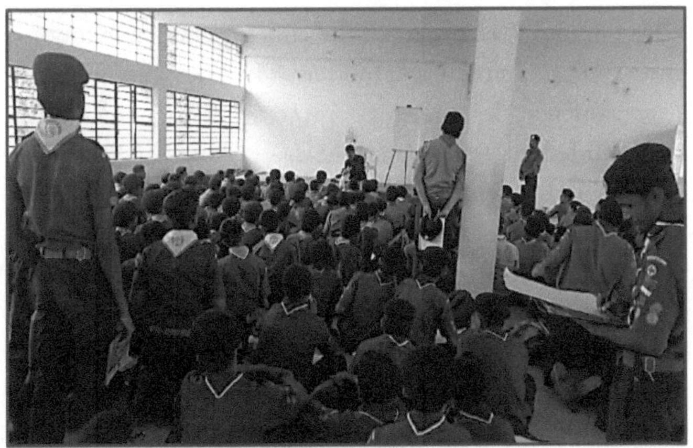

Training the school children and Teachers

Later, we gave first aid kits to all those police vans donated by Infosys. We also realized that even ordinary citizens could be empowered to handle common household emergencies. In order to achieve this, we expanded the curriculum and organized training sessions for senior citizens and homemakers in each locality.

This not only equipped them with essential life-saving skills but also enabled them to use their free time in a meaningful way by helping others in times of need.

That's when a new idea occurred to train school children and teachers. It was initiated primarily to manage their own emergencies. Secondly, during that period, there were a few serious accidents that happened, such as a

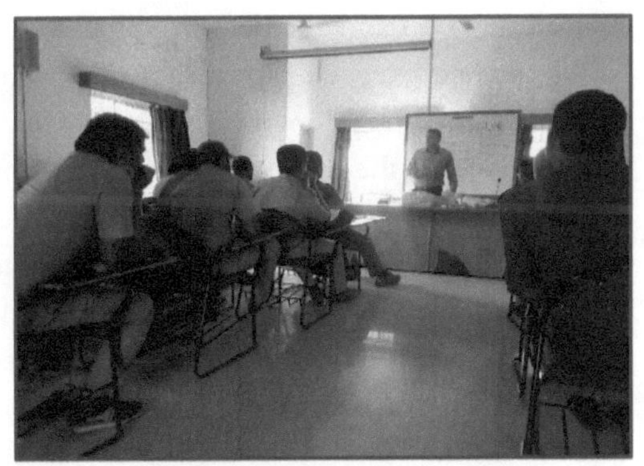

Training KSRTC Staff and Police in Basic First Aid

building collapse, a fire accident killing children in Tamil Nadu, and a terrorist attack on a school in Pakistan. All these prompted us to extend the training to all educational institutions.

By this time, we had mastered the entire training methodology and developed multiple structured modules. In line with our long-term vision, we launched the "PRIME" project – the Paramedic Research Institute for Medical Emergencies. Smt. Rohini Nilekani generously contributed ₹5 lakhs toward this school-based initiative. With these funds, we procured an additional projector and appointed dedicated trainers who traveled from school to school, conducting full-day sessions for classes 9 to 12.

The program quickly gained popularity and became highly sought after. Normally, when someone collapses on the road or an accident occurs, bystanders hesitate to help due to fear or misconceptions. Often, instead of assisting, people get into arguments or watch from the sidelines, or even worse, record the incident, leaving the injured person bleeding and unattended.

Maybe it's a little late for the older generation, but I believe that training children could change this mindset. We can teach them to become responsible Good Samaritans by instilling this value in them from a young age. Some might even choose to build a career in emergency medical care. Overall, the impact was remarkable.

Over 10 lakh students and several hundred teachers across Bangalore were trained under this initiative.

Meanwhile, several advancements were emerging in trauma management through ongoing research. However, these updates were not included in the standard curriculum, nor were any fundamental life-saving skills, such as CPR, are adequately emphasized in medical or nursing schools. This created a pressing need to train every medical and nursing student in these essential skills. To bridge this gap, we developed specialized training modules tailored for them. Participation was voluntary, and many students eagerly enrolled to receive this critical training. Meanwhile, we learned about an Australian-based program called CTLS (Comprehensive Trauma Life Support), which was being successfully implemented in Australia. They expressed willingness to conduct the course in India, and I reached out to Prof. Michel Parr from Sydney to make it happen. For the first time, we brought the CTLS course to Bangalore.

Since then, we have been conducting it annually for doctors and surgeons, equipping them with fundamental life-saving principles, practical skills, and updates on contemporary practices. Over the years, this initiative has enabled a large number of doctors to receive advanced trauma care training.

One of my ambitions was to create PRIME as a premier institution to take this forward. However, no one was clear about the jurisdiction under which the permissions could be obtained. I first approached Rajiv Gandhi University, but they said it doesn't come under their purview. The state government's paramedic board also stated that it can't give permission either. The definition of "paramedic" itself was unclear to the majority. To my disappointment, the entire project got stalled due to this confusion. The only option available was to affiliate with a foreign institution. That was possible, but it came with a huge cost which I wasn't able to afford at the time.

After several decades, skill labs finally became mandatory in medical colleges. Anticipating this need early on, we established the first skill station at Adi Chunchunagiri Medical College, thanks to the vision and support of the then chief pontiff, Maha Swamiji, Sri Dr. Balagangadharanatha Swamiji. Since then, the concept has evolved significantly, and the medical council has taken multiple steps to enhance emergency care training. However, pre-hospital care training remains an area that still requires substantial development.

Later, I collaborated with Washington University, and we initiated a 3-year course in emergency medicine. It had a well-defined syllabus, with faculty from the USA coming to teach at specified intervals, local faculty to guide students and supervise their skill sets, and finally, an exchange program that provided students with exposure in Washington. This provided them with the opportunity to learn from both countries' systems.

After conducting the course for five years, the Indian Medical Council introduced a local three-year MD program, which led us to discontinue the international hybrid course. We also approached the Ministry of Primary and Higher Education, advocating for the mandatory provision of emergency training for school children.

Despite several appeals, the proposal never materialized. Eventually, we designed a school safety program called *"Vidyarthi Suraksha"* and offered it voluntarily to various schools.

Vidyarthi Suraksha

The Program was specifically designed to ensure the safety of schools. Children, the future of our society, are highly vulnerable to threats and natural calamities. *Vidyarthi Suraksha* provides systematic guidelines for handling a wide range of situations, from minor injuries to major medical emergencies. It emphasizes strong infrastructure and preparedness, including emergency communication systems for contacting ambulances and police, training sessions for both students and teachers, safe evacuation procedures, designated assembly points, ambulance entry and rescue protocols, and efficient communication and tracking mechanisms. This comprehensive program not only provides knowledge but also empowers schools to become self-sufficient in preparing for and managing emergencies effectively. Many schools, particularly residential ones, came forward and implemented this training. Sri SA Chandran of the Essae Foundation provided constant support to all these programs and served as a mentor and a constant source of inspiration. He also provided the auditorium in his building at Koramangala for conducting training programs.

We had been using that as a standard location for training for quite some time. The availability of an equipped hall with a projector, screen, and teaching aids was very convenient for conducting training for various citizens.

Although these programs were very useful, the logistics of traveling to various locations with the team and all the teaching equipment became a challenge over time. To continue, we needed a massive scale-up of resources; otherwise, we would need to have a single institution where everyone comes and gets trained. So, finally, we established a proper training setup on the campus of Atria Institute of Engineering. Sri Chinna Swamy Raju kindly provided a location to set up a full-fledged training center with well-equipped classrooms and all the necessary teaching aids.

The center was inaugurated by Sri Chinnaswamy Raju himself. Even hostel facilities were offered to accommodate a few trainers, as well as those who plan to pursue this profession in the future. Although it was within the city, people began to complain about logistics, distance, and traffic, and the number of participants gradually dwindled.

EDU SAT Program of ISRO

Meanwhile, ISRO had developed a satellite-based education program, which was revolutionary at the time. It allowed large groups across the country to be trained simultaneously through satellite connectivity. From Bangalore, we could literally reach the entire nation. We took advantage of this opportunity by designing a program where all theoretical aspects would be delivered via satellite sessions. Later, we also planned to complement these with in-person contact programs for hands-on skill development, thereby creating a blended learning model.

This approach had the potential to become a massive nationwide initiative, establishing uniform standards for training across India. Initially, the program took off well, but over time, it failed to sustain. Eventually, even other similar educational programs declined and stopped altogether, forcing us to return to our original system and continue at a slower pace.

What began as a handful of white vans slowly grew into a movement that redefined pre-hospital care in our country. Every step, whether it was transforming ambulances into mobile ICUs, training paramedics and drivers to act as true lifesavers, establishing control rooms and tracking systems, or creating protocols for hospitals, was part of a larger vision to close the critical gap between accident and treatment. Along the way, we also broke new ground with the Green Corridor, experimented with air ambulances, and took training to schools, police, and ordinary citizens.

Additional Initiatives
1. Addressing the Challenge of Unknown Identity Cases
One of the most distressing challenges in trauma care is the problem of unknown identity. Following an accident, nearly 10% of patients are

admitted to hospitals as "unknown" cases, brought in by bystanders or the police, often unconscious and without any form of identification.

For their families, such situation is agonizing. When a loved one fails to return home, the search becomes a Herculean task, with no starting point and no clue whom to contact. Visiting every hospital is neither practical nor emotionally sustainable. In such cases, the police often take the lead in tracing family members, but this process can take two to three days or more. In those days, communication systems were limited, making the task even harder.

One particular incident highlighted the seriousness of this issue. A senior official from BHEL met with an accident on Old Madras Road and was admitted to a hospital by a good Samaritan. His family, unaware of his whereabouts, were in despair. In desperation, they contacted our CTC Control Room, hoping we might assist. Recognizing the urgency, our team immediately broadcast an alert through the police wireless network.

Within ten minutes, a hospital responded, confirming that such a person had been admitted with a head injury. The information was promptly relayed to his family, who were able to reach him without further delay.

This incident deeply reinforced the need for a structured communication link between hospitals, police, and the control room. We realized that timely information could save not only lives but also families from prolonged distress. From then on, we made it a policy to collect and update details of all "unknown" admissions across hospitals and assist families in tracing their loved ones.

What began as a single act of coordination eventually evolved into a social outreach initiative, one that bridged communication gaps and restored countless families during moments of crisis.

2. Health Centre at Kempegowda KSRTC Bus Station

The Kempegowda (Majestic) Bus Station in Bangalore often witnessed people suffering from various medical conditions and sometimes even dire emergencies. On average, three to five deaths occurred every month due to reasons ranging from exhaustion, dehydration, and long travel to seizures or other ailments.

Many people arriving in the city was already unwell, travelling from distant places to seek medical treatment, and would often collapse upon arrival.

The KSRTC authorities, who regularly handled such situations, reached out to us for support. They requested that we station an ambulance permanently at the bus terminal to handle these emergencies.

After reviewing the challenges and possibilities, we proposed a more comprehensive solution. Establishment of a dedicated medical Centre within the bus station itself. A space on the ground floor was allocated for this purpose. We equipped it with emergency drugs, a crash cart, a dressing room, and stationed an ambulance right outside for rapid response. MBBS doctors were appointed to provide round-the-clock medical care. Dr. Pramod took the lead in managing the center and ran it successfully for many years.

The facility proved to be a great support for both KSRTC employees and the general public. During the day, it functioned much like a primary health center, serving outpatients, while emergencies were promptly attended to and transferred to nearby hospitals. Many lives were saved, both at the bus station and at the adjacent City Railway Station.

We inaugurated the center in November 2004. After seeing the success of the center, when Mr. Muniappa became the railway minister, a similar center was established at Yeshwanthpur Railway Station, inaugurated by Sri Balagangadharanatha Mahaswamiji of Adichunchanagiri, at the Minister's request.

3. CTC – Suraksha

Patients arriving at emergency departments often face financial challenges. Accidents and injuries are never planned events, and most victims arrive without the means to pay for immediate treatment. At that time, medical insurance was still in its infancy, and existing policies rarely covered emergencies or injury-related expenses. Every patient required at least basic investigations, such as CT scans, and emergency procedures; however, the lack of funds frequently caused delays in treatment.

Often, victims were brought in by bystanders or police, who naturally could not take financial responsibility.

Even when relatives were present, they sometimes hesitated to give consent for treatment while debating the costs during those crucial first moments.

To address this persistent issue, we explored various approaches; however, none proved universally effective across hospitals. Eventually, we conceived the idea of introducing a specialized insurance scheme for accident victims. After extensive discussions with multiple insurers, New India Assurance Company agreed to collaborate on creating a customized accident policy named "CTC–Suraksha."

For an annual premium of ₹300, the policy offered ₹1 lakh coverage exclusively for accidents and injuries. Later, an optional air ambulance service was added for an additional ₹800 premium, making it one of the most comprehensive emergencies covers available at the time. However, selling the policy proved challenging. The public mindset was one of overconfidence, believing that accidents happen to others, not to oneself.

Despite our efforts and outreach, the uptake remained low, and the scheme eventually became unsustainable. Insurance systems depend on large volumes to remain viable, and the participation we anticipated never materialized.

4. Fundraising Event

Financial support was one of our greatest challenges. If we wanted to take our initiative to the level we aspired to be, without compromising on quality, resources were a must.

We needed resources for ambulances, medical equipment, Human Resources, continuous skill development, capacity building, expansions, quality control and monitoring services, all of which came with a cost. Initially, we all made personal contributions. Then support came from Mr S.A. Chandran of Essae Foundation, Mr Sundarraju of Atria, Mr SyamaRaju of Divyasree, Rotary, and others. Some companies started sponsoring the ambulance maintenance costs and providing various services. But building a sustainable model proved to be a major challenge for us.

We needed fundraising events. One such event was the S. P. Balasubrahmanyam concert. Mr Chandran, Mr Jagadish and Mr Gururaj came with me to meet Sri S.P. Balasubrahmanyam at the Kanteerava studio. We made a brief presentation, and he readily agreed to do a benefit musical programme and promised to support the organisation with such programmes every year. He was already supporting Thalassemia patients on a similar concept. As a team, we took responsibility for the entire event. Mr Gururaj, Jagdish, Paddy Menon, RT Kumar, and I formed the core team. Mr

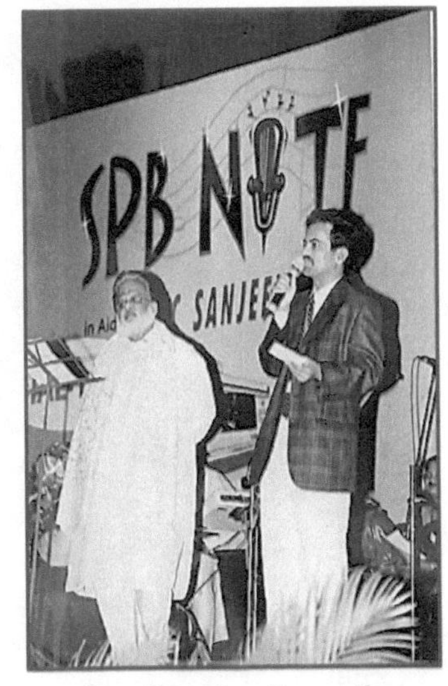

Fund Raising Concert by
SP Balasubrahmanyam

Syama Raju of Divyasree was the main sponsor. Mr Sunder Raju granted permission to use the KSLTA stadium for the event and helped with the arrangements. Radio city became an event partner and interviewed SPB for publicity.

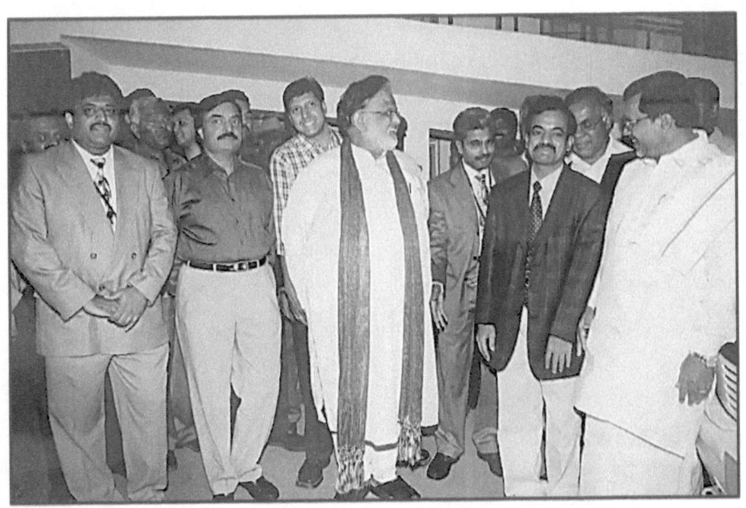

Arrival of Sri Siddaramaiah and Sri Sindhia for the inguaration
of the concert

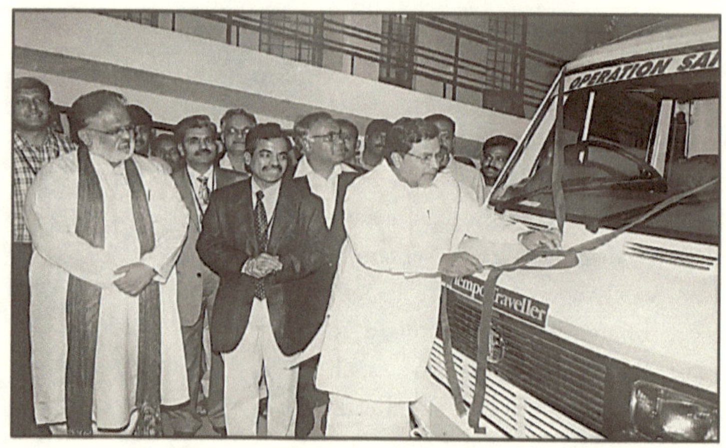

Inauguration of Ambulance Donated by Divyasree

The event was a huge success and lasted for three hours. Mr Siddaramaiah, the then finance minister and Mr PGR Scindhia were the main guests along with SPB.

The stadium was filled with people, and the money we received from the event could sustain the system for almost 9 months.

Looking back, we realize we were ahead of our time. Today, awareness has improved, and both personal and corporate insurance coverage have become more widespread. The importance of emergency and accident insurance is finally being understood, just as we had envisioned years ago. Each of these efforts came with its own share of obstacles, but with persistence, partnerships, and constant improvisation, we began to form a robust system.

The results spoke for themselves: lives were saved, deaths prevented, and an entire city becoming more aware and responsive in emergencies. More than just ambulances or equipment, it was about building trust, discipline, and a culture of responsibility.

This journey was far from complete. However, it had given us the courage to dream bigger and the clarity to see what the next chapter of emergency care in India could be.

CHAPTER – 5

Road Safety : A Culture We Forgot to Build

Transportation and Safety

Commuting has a long history, from walking on foot to flying. In the bargain, tremendous efforts have been made to make this process quick, safe, effective, and comfortable. When you think about it, out of all this, **safety** should be the one thing we guard the most. It must be the one goal that's researched, tested, implemented, and monitored without compromise. While every shiny innovation in transport has been eagerly embraced by industries, governments, and people alike, safety has somehow been left trailing behind. For all the progress we've made, the truth is, very little real effort or investment has gone into making our roads truly safe.

As a result, it continues to plague us for centuries. Transportation does not just involve roads and vehicles; it encompasses communication, safety, business, maintenance, innovation, research, implementation, enforcement, law, finance, quality control, suitable modifications, periodic upgrades, ongoing education, awareness, and constant monitoring, as well as good coordination. Sounds like a lot, doesn't it? But it's not, because the cost we're talking about here is human lives. Good roads without proper systems are no better than underdevelopment. Yes, we need effort in every area of transportation and infrastructure, but why is safety always the hardest to implement? It's almost paradoxical.

It is this strange, stubborn gap where everything else moves forward, yet safety lags behind. And the result?

We hold the grim record for the highest number of accidents and accident-related deaths in the world. In the end, good roads are more than just concrete and asphalt; they're a reflection of our culture, our systems, and our true progress.

Magnitude

India not only has the highest number of accidents, but it also lacks effective systems and a fundamental respect for safety. Creating a uniform transport system across the country requires effort and investment. Not just from the government's side, but also from the citizens' side. Following safety precautions costs nothing, yet somehow, we Indians are very hesitant about it. In fact, we relish in breaking rules.

I vividly remember the time I traveled to Geneva to attend a meeting with the WHO. My wife and daughter, who was very small at that time, were with me on the journey. We were traveling by train from Zurich to Geneva, and when we left the train station, it was getting late. There were only five taxis waiting in front of the station.

When they saw us, each of them came forward eagerly. The moment they saw my daughter, they hesitated. They said none of them have booster seats, which are essential for children under 150 cm in Geneva while traveling in vehicles.

They were willing to transport the suitcases and even my wife, but none of them agreed to take the child, even after I offered to pay more. In the end, my wife traveled with the luggage in a taxi, and I walked with my daughter for twenty minutes to join her at the hotel. Now, imagine this happening in India. We also have a law saying children under 135 cm should use a child restraint system while traveling, but it is rarely practiced.

No taxi driver is ever going to deny a ride under any circumstances. This is the difference our country has with other developed countries. There is a serious disregard for any rules. We seem to conveniently forget that these rules are there to preserve our lives.

Instead, we act like they are some huge inconveniences that are thrust upon us and take pride in breaking the rules.

As long as we cling to this mindset, no amount of advanced medical equipment is going to make a dent in our death toll. If the change in mindset doesn't happen, it reflects poorly on our culture. This single fact will negate all the other credibility.

The first recorded accident in the world occurred in Paris in 1771. In India, the first accident was reported in Kerala in 1914, taking the life of a prince of the Travancore royal family. From there, the number of accidents and deaths only ever increased. The Indian minds have become so immune to the news of deaths that no one cares or tries to make the system better. When all other countries have made phenomenal progress by keeping the numbers as low as possible, our country thrived on breaking the rules.

The result: the country is burdened with a huge number of deaths and the disabled year after year. The saddest part is that the highest number of deaths happens to people in the most productive age group of 15 to 35. Yet no one pays attention. Our population is our greatest resource, and yet, we treat it with a kind of casual negligence we can't afford. Every life lost or permanently disabled on the road is not just a personal tragedy; it is a blow to the country's economic strength and social fabric. The worst part? These deaths are not inevitable. They're preventable.

Road Traffic Accidents

Because of excessive speed, disorganized driving habits, and the constant rush, the number of road injuries keeps rising year after year, especially in developing countries like India. These accidents don't just affect drivers and passengers; they also put pedestrians at great risk of being hit by the crashing vehicles. The sad truth is that most of these incidents can be avoided if we remain vigilant, attentive, and responsible.

So, how do we prevent accidents? Where do we even begin? The answer is simple: start from the ground up. Literally, with the road itself.

The condition of the road plays a critical role in accident prevention. Cracks, potholes, slippery surfaces caused by rain, narrow lanes, poor-quality construction, inadequate signage, unscientific humps and barricades, and waterlogging are all potential hazards and recipes for disaster. Proper engineering and high-quality road construction are essential, along with identifying high-risk zones and implementing timely corrective measures.

Governments should build well-designed roads with smooth surfaces, scientifically calculated angles at curves, pothole-free stretches, standard speed-control measures such as approved humps or rumblers, properly designed shoulders, clear signage, and good visibility. In addition, strict enforcement of speed limits is also crucial. These factors collectively form the foundation for safer roads and fewer accidents.

The Science Behind Injury Prevention and Response

Medical specialists, biologists, and scientists have always been fascinated by the human body. Over time, the focus shifted to understanding its intricate systems and preserving their functions. The realization that the brain governs control, the heart pumps blood, the lungs exchange gases, the gut digests food with enzymes, the liver generates and stores energy, and the endocrine system regulates metabolism revealed the extraordinary complexity of our body. Along with this knowledge also came new challenges like diseases and injuries that continued to perplex and test human ingenuity.

Biochemistry and molecular biology have enabled us to understand the differential capabilities, abilities, sensitivities, and tolerance thresholds of each tissue. Thus, knowledge regarding the withstanding capacity of each tissue and cell to various possible threats came to light. Although every organ is susceptible, the brain appears to have the least tolerance, followed by the heart, the kidneys, and so on. This can indirectly determine the criticality and possibility of irreversible damage. Brain damage can directly correlate to death and disability. Therefore, damage prevention, tissue protection, and recovery promotion of the brain became the fundamental goal.

Continuous research, knowledge transformation, and advanced biotechnology have paved the way for the current understanding of this field.

As a result, the pathophysiology of the primary injury, as well as the subsequent serial changes, including inflammatory and immunological responses of the body, and their consequences, were deciphered over time.

1. Primary Prevention

"Prevention is better than cure" is not just a saying, but the ultimate truth when it comes to injuries. Instead of focusing on which hospital is better and which treatment you should get, you should be focusing more on avoiding the accident in the first place. Over the years, the focus has shifted toward designing safer roads, building better-engineered vehicles, introducing safety gadgets, and creating strict rules to enforce these measures. Among these, engineering has seen the most progress. Understanding the biomechanics of injuries, experts created experimental models to study the effects of head and spinal injuries. These models provided valuable insights, which in turn helped in developing various safety measures and gadgets.

However, here's the challenge: the forces involved in an impact are highly unpredictable. No single model can accurately capture the full range of real-world scenarios. Still, the knowledge gained from these models has been immensely helpful in making significant safety improvements. The real problem, though, is not the lack of safety solutions, but their adoption. Even when these measures have proven effective, they are not implemented consistently across the globe. In developing countries, especially, the mindset of people toward safety is still evolving. The shift toward prioritizing safety is underway, but it is happening slowly and unevenly.

2. Secondary Prevention

This approach is rooted in advanced medical understanding and focuses on preventing secondary injuries, the complications that occur after the initial trauma. **Primary injury** is the direct damage caused by the original impact, like a head injury or a fracture in an accident.

Secondary injuries, on the other hand, develop later due to delayed care, lack of oxygen, blood loss, or improper handling. These complications can be just as dangerous, sometimes even more so than the original injury, leading to death or lifelong disability.

The good news? Most secondary injuries can be controlled, or even avoided, if timely and proper intervention is provided. But time is critical. Action must be taken before the damage becomes irreversible. This understanding gave rise to the concept of the **"Golden Hour"**, the first crucial hour after an injury when prompt, appropriate action can save organs, preserve function, and minimize permanent damage.

The next big challenge was to bring all these right steps together in a proper sequence and ensure they work as a system. Perfecting this took time, but the results were worth the effort invested. Over the years, the concept evolved and became more structured and advanced, and is constantly scaling up. Now we have pre-hospital care, organized medical transportation, well-equipped ambulances, trained paramedics, emergency devices, and skill-based protocols. The progress is significant, but the true impact will only be realized when the entire system becomes uniform and standardized nationwide, and not just in Bangalore.

3. Tertiary Prevention

Tertiary prevention involves providing effective care to the patient when they reach the hospital and facilitating rehabilitation. The aim is to prevent all possible complications and to maximize tissue recovery. While the first two concepts minimize the extent of damage, the third one promotes recovery. Rehabilitation enhances functional recovery in order to restore the original ability.

A great deal has happened in this regard over the last few decades. Advances in imaging, monitoring, critical care, newer medications, clinical protocols, surgical techniques, and rehabilitation gadgets have made remarkable contributions to progress. All of these are being refined constantly through renewed learning and greater understanding. The current focus of pharmaceutical research is on tissue protection.

A significant amount of effort is being invested in tissue regeneration and tissue engineering to facilitate proper repair or replacement. Stem cell research holds great promise for repairing or restoring brain function, although it presents several challenges to overcome.

The Impact of Timely Intervention

The benefits of timely intervention are not limited to trauma care—they extend across a wide range of medical emergencies.

Over time, this principle of acting fast has proven life-saving in conditions such as:

- Spinal injury
- Heart attack
- Brain stroke
- Vascular injuries
- Bleeding
- Shock
- Reimplantation of injured and amputated parts of the body

These examples demonstrate how the concept of the **Golden Hour** has evolved beyond trauma care to become a universal guideline for critical medical situations. The key idea remains the same. There is a time-sensitive window where, with the right actions, damage can be reversed and life can be saved. This window varies depending on the condition, but the urgency never changes. For instance: In severe brain injuries, the first hour remains absolutely critical. For ischemic stroke, the "golden period" extends to approximately 3 to 4.5 hours, during which clot-busting drugs (thrombolysis) can be effective. In heart attacks, opening the blocked artery with stenting or thrombolysis within 90 minutes saves the heart muscle.

This evolving understanding gave rise to modern emergency interventions, including:

- **Thrombolysis** for stroke and heart attack – dissolving blood clots before they destroy brain or heart tissue.
- **Emergency stenting** – opening blocked arteries to restore circulation.
- **Early brain surgery** – to remove clots, stop hemorrhage, or repair aneurysms.
- **Arterial embolization** – to control internal bleeding and prevent shock.

- **Vascular reconstruction** – to repair or replace damaged blood vessels.
- **Microsurgical reimplantation** – to restore amputated parts before they die from lack of blood supply.

All these techniques share a common thread: time is the deciding factor between life, disability, and death. Research evidence and clinical experience have shaped clear protocols and streamlined medical practices to ensure no second is wasted.

Over the years, the Golden Hour evolved into a series of condition-specific timelines that guide doctors, paramedics, and systems to act with precision and speed. The earlier we act, the better the outcome. Every minute counts.

Brain Attack

No one needs to be taught about the emergency of a heart attack. It happens when the blood flow to the coronary arteries in the heart is reduced or blocked, preventing oxygen from reaching the heart and damaging the heart muscles. If emergency medical care is not sought, a heart attack can result in the patient's demise. A brain attack is a similar medical condition that is as important as a heart attack, and one that people need to be more aware of. A brain attack or stroke occurs when blood flow to the brain is interrupted or a blood vessel in the brain ruptures, causing brain cell death. Both conditions affect the vital organs of the body and are caused by disruptions in blood circulation.

During a brain stroke, when the blood supply is blocked or reduced, it deprives the brain tissue of oxygen and essential nutrients, which causes brain cells to die. There are two main types of brain stroke: ischemic stroke, caused by a blockage in a blood vessel, and hemorrhagic stroke, caused by a ruptured blood vessel. The brain is highly sensitive to even brief interruptions in blood flow, and depending on the area affected, a stroke can result in weakness or paralysis, difficulty speaking, vision problems, loss of balance, or even memory and cognitive decline. Since the brain controls all bodily functions, the effects of a stroke can be widespread and often permanent, making it one of the leading causes of disability and death worldwide.

Early recognition and immediate treatment are critical to limit brain damage and improve recovery.

The Golden Hours for Brain Attack

The symptoms of a brain attack include face drooping or numbness, Arm weakness or inability to lift both arms, or difficulty in speaking or slurred speech. If any of these symptoms are experienced, you must call emergency services without delay. Just like a heart attack, time is very crucial for a brain attack. You cannot ignore it or wait in a queue for hours and treat it like a cold or a fever. Brain cells have a set amount of tolerance, which is **three hours**. If, within these three hours, the nutrition and oxygen are restored through the blood supply, the brain can be revived. This is the golden hours of a brain attack. If we fail to act within the golden hours, it is almost guaranteed that there will be a certain amount of brain damage. Unfortunately, due to a lack of awareness among citizens in our country, many believe it is not necessary to rush to the hospital. Therefore, in the majority of situations, the golden hours are missed, and the patient either dies or suffers permanent disability.

Treatment

Brain stroke is treated by focusing on restoring the blood flow to the brain as quickly as possible to prevent any lasting damage. The immediate care involves timely diagnosis, quick initiation of treatment, and interventions to remove or dissolve blockages in blood vessels. Early restoration of blood circulation reduces brain damage and improves recovery outcomes. It is also crucial that proper care is taken to protect the affected area, monitor for complications such as swelling or seizures, and provide intensive care when needed. There is also long-term treatment for brain stroke patients, like rehabilitation and managing risk factors to prevent future strokes. A brain attack has several risk factors. These include physical factors like obesity, sedentary lifestyle, smoking, and sleep disorders, as well as biochemical conditions such as diabetes, hypertension, and lipid abnormalities.

Other diseases, such as heart and kidney problems, autoimmune disorders, malignancies, and metabolic conditions, also increase the risk. People with uncontrolled diabetes or hypertension, blood or inflammatory disorders, cardiac arrhythmias, or a family history of stroke or heart attack belong to the high-risk group and require close monitoring.

If we are careful enough, we can prevent the possibility of having a stroke.

Primary prevention

- Regular health checks
- Healthy living
- Emotional well-being
- Vigilant monitoring,

Secondary prevention

- Strict adherence to treatment
- Regular follow-ups
- Modification of risk factors
- Continuous vigilance to prevent recurrence.
- Emotional well-being

Complications of a Brain Attack

If not treated in time, the complications of a brain attack can be devastating, ranging from pain and deformity to long-term disability and even death. The severity depends on several factors, such as the type of stroke, the patient's age, the time when treatment is initiated, and the support systems available to them. Often, the damage affects more than the patient. In cases of disability like loss of speech, memory, vision, or paralysis, the patient becomes completely dependent on others. Without proper therapy, frozen joints, muscle wasting, and deformities can set in, worsening the situation.

The emotional burden a stroke can bring is also equally harsh. The loss of independence, unemployment, and social isolation often push patients into depression. This situation also affects the families of patients.

If the main earning member suffers a stroke, it can plunge the entire household into financial and emotional crisis. This is why you must take the condition seriously and seek treatment within the golden hours.

According to statistics, in our country, nearly 180 to 210 people per lakh suffer a stroke, and every year, around two million new cases are added to the list. The tragedy is that the numbers are not entirely accurate due to the lack of clarity in our systems. What we have is only an estimate. Compare this with the United States, where over 795,000 people suffer a stroke annually, and where the impact is studied, documented, and addressed with seriousness. The World Health Organization estimates that around 15 million people worldwide are struck by ischemic stroke each year, with several million losing their lives or living with lifelong disability.

The economic burden is equally frightening. Globally, the management of stroke drains around 184 billion dollars annually, but in India, we have little understanding of the true financial loss, especially the long-term costs of disability and treatment. When the main earning member of a family is hit by a stroke, it is not just a medical crisis; it shakes the very foundation of the household. Abroad, social support systems are structured to soften the blow, but here, families are left to struggle alone. Until we address this gap with honesty and commitment, the so-called "burden of stroke" will only keep growing heavier on our people and our nation.

Heart Attack

A heart attack, medically known as a *myocardial infarction*, occurs when the blood supply to part of the heart muscle is reduced or blocked, causing damage to the heart. This is a medical emergency in which every second counts.

When to Suspect a Heart Attack

- Assume a heart attack if someone is showing any of the following signs:
- Chest pain or discomfort that feels like pressure, squeezing, tightness, or aching.

- Pain or discomfort spreading to the shoulder, arm, back, neck, jaw, teeth, or upper belly.
- Shortness of breath, light-headedness, or sudden dizziness.
- Cold sweats, nausea, a heartburn-like feeling, and fatigue.
- Note: In some individuals, particularly women, the symptoms may be milder or less noticeable.

What to Do Immediately

- Call emergency services without delay.
- If instructed by a medical professional, give aspirin (which helps prevent blood clotting) but only after calling for help.
- If the person has a prescribed nitroglycerin for heart conditions and is aware it's for them, administer it as directed while waiting for help.
- If the person is unconscious or not breathing normally, start CPR (if trained). If not trained, do hands-only chest compressions (~100-120 per minute) until professional help arrives.
- If an AED (automated external defibrillator) is available and the person is unconscious, use it as instructed.

Why Timely Action Is Critical

Every minute of delay allows more of the heart muscle to become damaged. The faster the blood flow is restored, the better the chances of survival and recovery. Ignoring symptoms or waiting too long can lead to irreversible heart damage, heart failure, or death.

Basic Prevention Tips

- Healthy choices reduce the risk of a heart attack. Key habits include:
- Don't smoke, and avoid tobacco use.
- Engage in regular physical activity.
- Maintain a healthy weight, eat nutritiously (less salt, less saturated fat).

- Limit alcohol intake; manage stress.
- Monitor and control blood pressure, blood sugar and cholesterol.
- Ensure adequate sleep (7-8 hours) each night.
- Consider getting trained in CPR and the use of AEDs to be ready to help others.

Spinal Injury

A spinal injury is one of the most serious and potentially life-changing types of traumas a person can suffer. The spinal cord controls movement, sensation, and numerous vital bodily functions. Any damage to it can result in permanent paralysis, loss of sensation, or, in extreme cases, even death. They are more common than most people realize, often resulting from road accidents, falls, sports injuries, or workplace incidents. Even a seemingly minor mishandling of an injured person can worsen the damage and lead to irreversible complications. Therefore, knowing what to do and what not to do in such situations is extremely important.

When to Suspect a Spinal Injury

- Always assume a spinal injury in the following situations:
- The person is unconscious or unresponsive.
- The person complains of severe pain in the neck or back.
- There is weakness, numbness, paralysis, or loss of control over limbs or bladder.
- The neck, back, or body appears twisted, or the posture looks abnormal.

What to Do if You Suspect a Spinal Injury

- **Call for help immediately.** Dial emergency services and alert people nearby for assistance.
- **Keep the person still.** Do not attempt to move them unless absolutely necessary for safety.

- **Stabilize the head and neck.** Use rolled towels or sheets on either side, or hold them firmly to prevent any movement.
- **Do not remove a helmet** unless it obstructs breathing.
- **Never move the person alone.** At least four people are required to safely lift a spinal injury victim: One person supports the head and neck, keeping them in a straight line with the spine. One supports the upper chest. One supports the pelvis. One holds the legs together. The person should be lifted carefully onto a spinal board or hard surface, maintaining alignment at all times.

Common Causes of Spinal Injury

- Falls from height.
- Sports or gymnastics accidents, especially awkward landings.
- Diving into shallow water and hitting the bottom.
- Motorbike or vehicle accidents, especially with sudden deceleration.
- Heavy objects falling on the back.
- High-speed head or facial trauma.

Signs and Symptoms

- Look for the following warning signs:
- Severe pain in the neck or back at the injury site.
- Abnormal shape or twist in the spine's normal curve.
- Tenderness, bruising, or discoloration over the spine.
- Weakness or loss of movement in arms or legs.
- Loss or alteration of sensation, such as tingling or numbness.
- Difficulty or inability to pass urine.
- Breathing difficulties or irregular breathing.

Why Timely Action Matters

Delay or mishandling in spinal injury cases can make the difference between full recovery and lifelong disability.

Even a single wrong movement can worsen the injury, leading to irreversible spinal cord damage. Prompt medical attention, immobilization, and transport to a hospital with trauma care facilities are essential to improving outcomes.

Keeping Pace with Medical Progress

Nowadays, medical science is advancing at an incredible pace and is introducing new treatments while continually refining and validating existing methods. In times like these, the concept of the Golden Hour has become increasingly important, extending far beyond trauma care to include a wide range of medical emergencies.

However, progress comes with a dual challenge. On one hand, keeping up with the latest developments, and on the other hand, implementing them effectively from the ground up. Striking this balance is critical. If we adopt everything at once without proper structure, the system becomes chaotic. If we do nothing, we remain stagnant. Both extremes will lead to failure.

The solution for these issues is sustained effort and continuous focus. We need to update medical practices step by step while ensuring they are practical, accessible, and in a standardized form. This is particularly crucial in emergencies, where the initial response often relies on locally available resources. No matter how advanced medical science becomes, it is the timely application of available tools and systems that determines the outcome in those critical moments.

Following Road Rules

Regardless of the road one is travelling, the rules must be followed without any modifications or compromise. In fact, it is becoming a challenge for the traffic police to achieve this, especially in cities where the concept of civic responsibility is increasingly being disregarded.

A significant amount of manpower is being wasted solely to monitor this single task. If everyone is disciplined, the police force can be used effectively elsewhere for a better purpose. Unfortunately, they are also toiling day and night, standing in the adverse weather and pollution just to control the citizens' driving practices.

No other country does this. Civic attitudes don't require supervision; only then can they be called self-discipline.

The basic rules must be well-versed by every driver, regardless of the vehicle they are driving. Drivers should always maintain lane discipline, avoid unnecessary overtaking, keep a safe distance between vehicles, and respect pedestrians and zebra crossings. You should also obey traffic signals regardless of the time of day or how empty the road appears. It is not optional. Jumping the signal, overtaking on the wrong side, confusing other drivers on the road, travelling opposite on a one-way street, stopping at inappropriate places, or parking haphazardly should be avoided at all costs. Safe driving is not just a personal choice, nor is it for the benefit of the government. It is a social obligation, and more than that, it is for your own safety.

The licensing system also requires strict reform to ensure that only qualified and trained drivers are on the road. As responsible citizens, we must discourage untrained and reckless driving. Additionally, the increasing chaos caused by two-wheelers needs special attention. A dedicated lane for two-wheelers will reduce the risk of collisions and streamline traffic flow.

Right now, their unpredictable movement is almost like the mosquito menace; everywhere, buzzing in and out, and creating hazards for everyone.

Road Safety Precautions

1. Helmet

Undoubtedly, the helmet prevents head injury. The impact on the head will be reduced by 50% if you are wearing a helmet. There are enough studies and evidence to suggest that helmets reduce the incidence of skull fractures, severity of brain injury, and blood clots in the brain.

Many have the wrong idea about helmets. A proper standard, ISI-marked, full-face helmet is beneficial.

Proper size and strapping are essential for complete protection. Your brain is a vital organ, and you must be responsible for protecting it. Don't wear it for the sake of the police.

It is also recommended for the pillion rider. Often, the pillion sustains more serious injuries than the rider. One should not avoid it on the pretext of weight, hair loss, hairstyle distortion, or interference with hearing. Having a healthy head is more important than all these.

2. Seat Belt

A seat belt is a game-changer in preventing spine injuries. In a high-speed vehicle, the sudden cessation of movement can cause a variety of jerky and rotational movements that are hazardous to the body tissues, particularly the brain and spine. This sudden forward-backward movement can cause subluxation or dislocation of the spinal bones or whiplash injury to the spine, causing paralysis of the limbs.

Wearing a seatbelt properly can avoid this complication entirely. It is recommended to wear a belt, even on city roads, and for short distances. Most cars have alarm systems for those who are in the front seats. But it is essential to wear them even in the back seats. On many occasions, people were thrown out of cars, negating the built-in safety systems by not wearing seatbelts.

3. Vehicle Conditions

The standards of vehicles and automobile engineering are constantly advancing. A substantial amount of research has been conducted in this area. Many new systems, alarms, crash zones, airbags, and safety devices are incorporated in the building of every vehicle. Fortunately, many such good cars are now available in our country.

Apart from buying a vehicle, good maintenance, servicing, and timely replacement of worn-out parts, such as brake pads, wheel discs, and tires, are also important.

Outdated vehicles must be disposed of, and fitness certification must be rigorous.

4. Adverse Situations

Even if you have a good vehicle and follow all safety precautions, there are still factors that remain beyond your control. Geographical terrain and unpredictable weather conditions are two major ones. Drivers must always be aware of these variables and stay prepared for sudden changes.

During winter fogs, visibility drops drastically, making it impossible to see the road clearly. This increases the chance of getting into an accident.

In such cases, using fog lights, reflectors, proper signage, and strict speed control can be helpful, along with the driver's experience and judgment. Similarly, heavy rain and flooding can turn roads into dangerous traps.

Waterlogging hides potholes, reduces friction, and increases the risk of skidding or hydroplaning. Flash floods can completely block roads or even sweep vehicles away.

The safest approach is to slow down, maintain extra distance, avoid sudden braking, and never attempt to cross a flooded stretch without first assessing its depth and current.

Driving Hygiene and Personal Habits

1. Sleep

Drivers should avoid overworking, as lack of sleep reduces alertness and judgment. Sleep needs vary, but listen to your body and rest when you need to. For overnight drivers, this is even more critical. Drowsy driving can be as dangerous as drunk driving. If you feel sleepy, stop and take a break.

2. Food

Similarly, food is very important, particularly for those who are diabetic. The diet schedule should be very strict. Overeating is not at all advisable. Food should be light yet sufficient to meet the body's needs for sufficient energy. The quality of food is also important. Oily foods, curd rice, and heavy sweets can induce sleep while driving.

3. Water

Drinking adequate water is beneficial, especially in hot environments. People who are accustomed to coffee or tea can have them. Again, excess is not advisable. Drinking cold water as well as washing the face frequently is preferable.

Avoid Substances that Impair Judgment

1. Alcohol

Alcohol while driving must be avoided at any cost. Regardless of the volume of alcohol consumed, it can cause significant problems.

Apart from long-term health issues, it can alter brain activity. The brain can become dull, sleepy, and judgment will be compromised. One can either become overconfident or unable to make the right decisions. Both can have serious consequences, including accidents. You have to be careful about other drunken drivers on the road, also. Even if you aren't the one who is drunk, you still can get injured due to others' mistakes.

2. Smoking

Many think that smoking stimulates the brain, hence they resort to it. In reality, it is quite misleading. No doubt it provides some stimulation to the brain.

However, it is short-lived, and subsequent doses can be highly detrimental. Long-term smoking or tobacco chewing can lead to high BP, cancer, stroke, and a variety of toxic effects on many organs.

3. Avoid All Distractions

It is essential to train drivers to avoid all possible distractions. Even a momentary loss of attention can lead to dangerous problems. Often, these distractions are the cause of accidents, particularly on highways and at high speeds. Mobile phones, TV, movies, loud radio noise, distractions from others in the vehicle, adjusting the seat position or steering position, drinking water, or eating can cause the driver to lose focus and the vehicle to lose control at high speeds.

One must avoid them as much as possible, and if you have to give your attention to something else, it should be done when the vehicle is parked at a safe place.

4. Mental Status

A good mental state is essential for safe driving, as well as for effective day-to-day work. A disturbed mental state for any reason can affect attention, judgment, and often cause confusion. A balanced state of mind can be of great assistance directly or indirectly.

One should avoid driving in a disturbed state of mind, such as after a fight or other emotional stress.

Road safety is not just about rules, vehicles, or infrastructure; it is also about building a culture of responsibility and respect for human life, which we Indians lack. Every time an accident is avoided, a life is saved, and precaution is taken, it reflects the value we place on ourselves and others. There is no point in reading through all these steps if you are not willing to practice them. Change should begin with each one of us. If we truly wish to progress as a nation, we must build a culture where safety is not an afterthought but the foundation of every journey.

CHAPTER – 6

Innovations on Wheels

Highway Culture

A highway is a main public road designed for fast and long-distance travel, typically connecting cities, towns, or states. It has multiple lanes, controlled access, and minimal intersections to facilitate smooth traffic flow.

The concept of highways dates back thousands of years, evolving from basic dirt paths during the Mesopotamian and Egyptian civilizations to the modern expressways we have today. Though it had its ups and downs, by the 17th and 18th centuries, the rise in trade and commerce also increased the demand for better roads. With the invention of the automobile in the 20th century, asphalt and concrete highways became standard. The first ever automobile-only road was built in 1921 in Germany. They are called *Autobahns*. They were built with impressive engineering knowledge and became famous for their quality and stability. In fact, when Adolf Hitler came to power in 1933, he accelerated the Autobahn project as part of his efforts to create jobs and boost national pride. I had the fortune of traveling on those roads while I was in Germany.

People will travel at 200 to 250 kilometers per hour at times. Despite the speed, the number of accidents is so meager. The reason for the low number was the civic responsibility of the citizens. Everyone follows the system, obeys the rules, and no one ever tries to break the rules. The cultural difference was obvious. People prefer to go by road rather than by flight in those countries.

I recall once traveling from Frankfurt to Berlin and arriving earlier than expected. The roads were so smooth and well-maintained that the journey was not just convenient but also an absolute pleasure.

Roads indicate civilization and culture. Although our country does not have a strong history of high-quality roads, things are changing for the better. Road infrastructure is improving, and modern expressways are being developed nationwide. Expressways will have several lanes and will have different etiquette, systems, and rules to follow without any compromise. Unfortunately, the driving culture in India is so chaotic that even on highways, many continue with the same reckless habits. Driving on a high-speed expressway is a completely different experience. It's not a football match where vehicles can dart around in a zigzag manner; It demands discipline.

Fundamentally, an expressway must follow certain key standards. It should provide a smooth, uninterrupted ride without surprises, obstacles, or hindrances. Local authorities or individuals should not alter the design or add unauthorized features to the structure. Internationally accepted norms strictly prohibit speed breakers, humps, barricades, or random checkpoints on expressways. There should be no direct crossovers from side roads; access is only through designated interchanges. Stray animals and pedestrians are strictly barred, and hawkers or unauthorized vendors are not permitted under any circumstances.

The expressway has a lane culture. Lanes and all signage, including speed limits, should be clearly visible. The two-wheelers must stay on the extreme left. Heavy vehicles such as buses and trucks will occupy the next left lanes. Only the fast-moving vehicles will stay on the right lanes. No overtaking from the left is allowed. Overtaking and lane changing must be done in a systematic manner, using proper indicators, and only when the lane is clear of other vehicles. No sudden stopping of vehicles is allowed except in a designated place in an emergency. The designated speeds must be followed strictly, and drivers must be well-adapted and trained before they drive on such highways.

Unfortunately, many Indian drivers are unaware of the rules and discipline on highways, particularly taxi and truck drivers.

Therefore, we need to strengthen the system in such a way that all drivers are aware of it and have sufficient knowledge. For that, we must first make our licensing system more scientific and rigorous.

Secondly, all highways should have emergency speed-detecting cameras, emergency telephonic access at regular intervals, and a display of emergency helplines. Highway hospitals must be equipped to handle any emergencies. When planning such a project, provisions for the ambulance bay, first aid center, and helipads must be designated. So, one needs to be educated in all these aspects and the highway ecosystem. Police patrolling expressways must be extremely strict to ensure compliance with all these rules and regulations.

Highway Trauma Care

Bangalore had five arterial highways connecting to various parts of the city. Each highway in those days had its own unique characteristics and challenges, with accident-prone areas and a high number of casualties. They include old Madras Road, Mysore Road, Bellary Road, Tumkur Road, and Hosur Road. Among them, the old Madras Road and Mysore Road had the highest number of accidents, followed by Tumkur Road.

After examining the numbers, we considered creating a system to make these highways safer for vehicles and civilians.

We first targeted hospitals already situated near the highway and equipped them with the latest medical instruments, training their professionals accordingly. A good friend and very active philanthropic doctor, Dr. Nagaraj, had a hospital at Hosakote called Srinivasa Hospital, which provided significant support to the old Madras Road. He even organized several training programs and awareness programs for the hospitals and the public in the highway region. A dedicated, well-equipped ambulance was also kept ready for emergencies in strategic locations.

We talked with the police and identified the most accident-prone areas on these highways. Each of those locations presented its own logistical challenges, making it hazardous for vehicles. However, one common factor that stood out was the complete lack of any medical facilities nearby. This meant that arranging an ambulance or any form of emergency response was nearly impossible. On highways, the chances of a passerby stepping in to help are also slim, leaving victims with little to no immediate assistance. This insight drove us to design an entirely different model from what was used in the city. We needed a system that could provide readily accessible help at all times.

The new highway emergency model was built on the same core principles of communication, transportation, and immediate care, with an enhanced approach.

The old concept of "grab and go" was no longer effective. Instead, the focus shifted to assessing and stabilizing the patient first before transferring them to the vehicle. We trained the drivers and paramedics in all the necessary techniques and knowledge, so that they could ensure a clear airway, proper breathing, and adequate circulation before moving them. This strategy buys crucial time and allows for safe transport to the appropriate hospital.

We also stationed ambulances and established first-aid centers along the highways to provide immediate resuscitation whenever necessary.

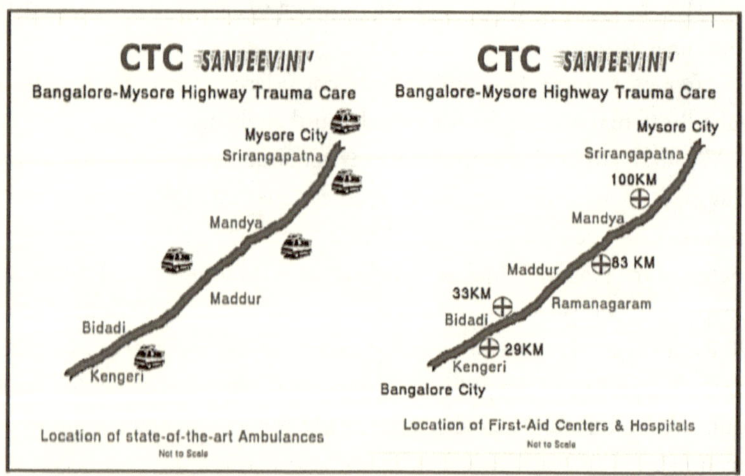

Bangalore-Mysore Highway Trauma Care

The Comprehensive Trauma Consortium ensured an ambulance station every 25 km; a system ahead of its time. Unfortunately, that entire network has now become obsolete. Unless we rebuild and modernize this system, true highway safety will remain a distant dream. On every expressway, safety, not speed, must be the top priority. Only then can we aspire to match the standards of developed nations.

The Mysuru–Bengaluru expressway is undoubtedly a laudable and much-needed project. However, it is deeply concerning that the number of accidents and fatalities surged soon after its inauguration. Similar patterns have been observed with almost every bypass and ring road in the past. We must adopt international best practices, not just in road construction but, more importantly, in transforming our driving culture and mindset. All stakeholders, including government bodies, enforcement agencies, and road users, are required to implement and adhere to these safety guidelines without any compromise. This will ensure that our roads are not only faster but also truly safe and purposeful.

Placement of the Ambulance

Stationing an ambulance at a strategic location is crucial. An ambulance must be able to reach the patient, retrieve them, and transport them to the hospital before the golden hour expires. However, it is far easier to do this when a medical facility is nearby.

However, that is not the case on highways. It takes a long time to reach back to towns and villages if the accident occurs in the middle of the highway. This was why we came up with the idea of parking ambulances at fuel stations. Fuel stations are open 24 hours, making it easy to get help at all times.

We presented this idea to Indian Oil in a meeting held at the office of my friend, Mr. Ramamohan Reddy. After several meetings, permission was obtained for three locations: Mysore Road, Narasapura on the Bangalore-Chennai highway, and Dabaspet on the Tumkur highway, all of which are company outlets. We first initiated a trial at these sites. Ambulances with trained paramedics were stationed at two of these locations.

We even gave the petrol station employees first aid training so that they can provide assistance if required. Dr. Prasanna and Dr. Satish helped us in providing the training to the employees.

The concept is simple: in the event of an accident or medical emergency on the highway, individuals can rush to the nearest petrol station for help, emergency medications, and, if necessary, ambulance transport to the hospital. While these new arrangements were being made, we decided to undertake a proper project on Mysore Road. By then, we had acquired a few more ambulances, which were donated by Divyasree, the Embassy, and other corporations. We reshuffled them and placed five ambulances between Bangalore and Mysore. The distance between the two cities is 125 kilometers. So, every 25 Km, an ambulance was placed. The exact locations were chosen based on accident statistics and high-risk areas rather than geography. Our goal was to connect them via wireless for seamless communication. We identified high-power wireless stations on Chamundi Hills and, after coordinating with the authorities in Mysore and Bangalore, established connectivity between Chamundi Hills and the Utility Building on MG Road.

Several technical challenges arose in capturing accurate signals and ensuring each ambulance network met the required standards.

Mr. Rajaram invested significant effort to overcome these challenges. Initially, we lacked some equipment and boosters, but fortunately, Mr. Chandrasekahar Raju of Sri Chamaraju Kalyan Mandap

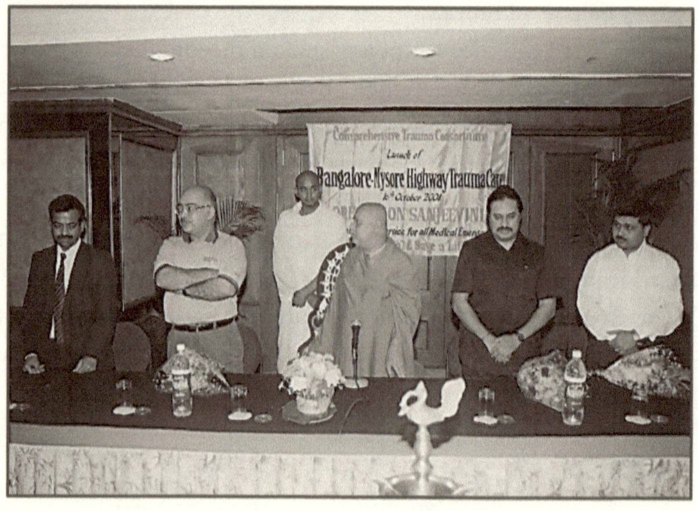

Inauguration of Bangalore- Mysore Highway Trauma Project

generously provided the necessary equipment, enabling us to successfully create the wireless network. The Bangalore-Mysore highway project was officially launched on 10 October 2004 by Sri Sri Balagangadharanatha Mahaswamiji of the Adichunchanagiri Mutt. The launch was successfully held at Hotel Atria, Bangalore.

Solar-Powered First-Aid Centers

With CTC and Golden hour, what I envisioned was a revolutionary change in emergency medical care. However, no such vast-scale change has ever been accomplished alone. I received help from various industry experts and government officials throughout the journey. One such impactful collaboration was with Mr. Satpati of Tata BP Solar. Mr. Satpati was always an enthusiast of innovative projects and a dynamic, forward-looking person. They had an office at Electronic City. After listening to our concept, he came up with the idea of solar-powered stations. We held several rounds of discussions and eventually agreed to develop a model powered entirely by solar energy.

The solar panels would serve as the primary power source and would run all essential equipment, lighting, and monitors seamlessly. My team and I, along with Mr. Satpati, sat down and calculated all the equipment that should be included in this, and reworked the requirements for solar panels and batteries.

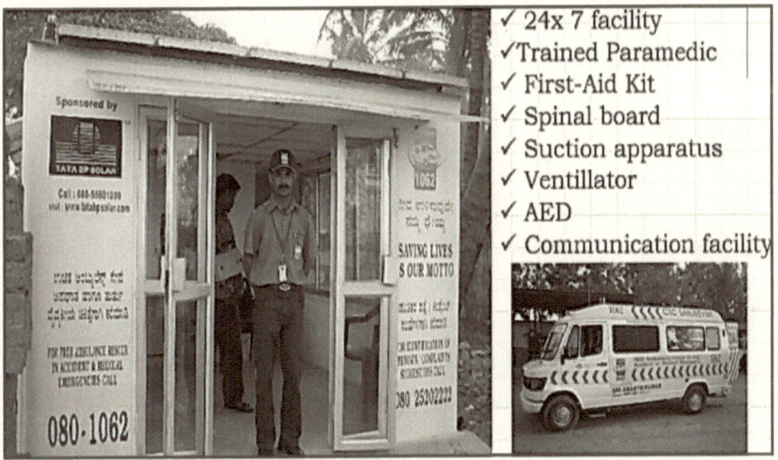

Solar-Powered First-Aid Centers on Mysore Road

Then Mr. Satpathi came up with the idea of building the stations with lightweight, fabricated walls and a floor for efficiency.

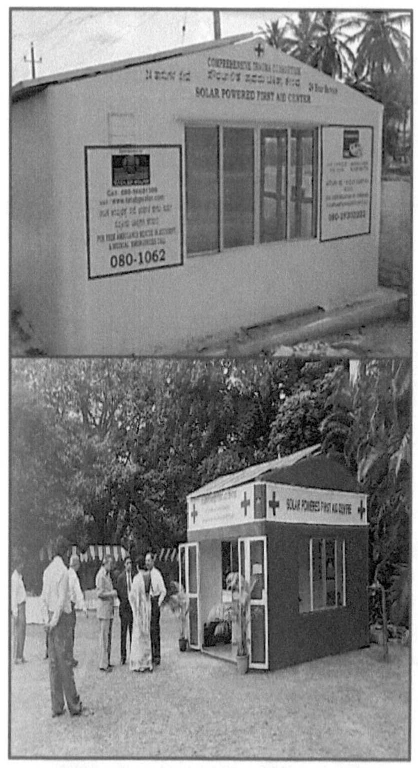

Models of Solar Powered First Aid Centers

The idea was simple yet powerful. Set up life-saving centers at key points along the highway, each fully equipped and ready to function as an independent emergency unit. These centers would house all essential equipment like wireless communication devices, computers, patient monitors, transport ventilators, automated external defibrillators (AEDs), powered suction units, and adequate lighting. A trained paramedic would be present at each station to conduct initial assessments, stabilization, and resuscitation as necessary. To make the model sustainable and efficient, every piece of equipment would run on solar energy. From charging devices to powering lights and medical systems, solar power will be the backbone of these stations.

The advantages of this model were clear. These units can be installed exactly where needed within a short amount of time, with an ambulance stationed right beside them. If the highway were widened or the location became unsuitable for any reason, the entire setup could be easily relocated. To bring this idea to life, we needed a prototype, and Mr. Satpati and his team delivered it in record time. We were excited to showcase this innovation and decided to do a demonstration. We arranged a complete setup with all the necessary equipment inside and even simulated a real rescue mission using mannequins.

Our audience was none other than Sri Ratan Tata himself, who listened attentively as I explained the concept and watched the demo with keen interest.

After the demo, he not only appreciated the idea but was also kind enough to sanction the establishment of 50 such centers for the organization.

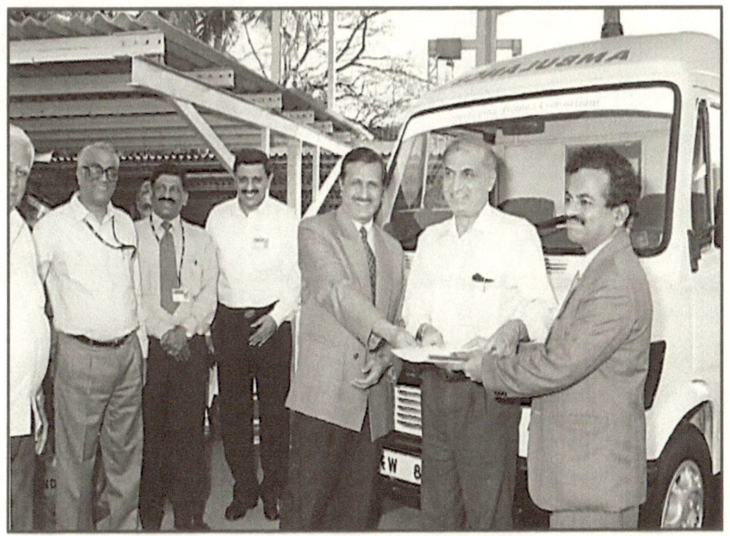

Donation of Ambulance by MICO With Sri Lakshminarayana and Sri Madiyal

That moment was a milestone and a proud achievement for both CTC and Tata BP Solar. It proved that a bold idea, backed by innovation and commitment, can truly transform lives.

Once we received the signal to proceed with our stations, the next task was to place them on the sides of the highways.

We needed land and some form of security to protect the people and equipment. Our first choice was the Indian Highway Authority.

We appealed for permission to both the Bangalore office and the central office. Since it was taking a long time, we also approached a few landowners with land on the roadside to lend us a small space.

However, it was difficult to convince many. Even the swamiji of Viswa Vokkaligara Sangha, located on the Mysore Road, refused to help.

We had to meet several people and explain the concept. When some gave time-bound permission, stating that this should be removed after three months, others put their demands. With the help of some good Samaritans who agreed to host them, we were able to place them in reasonably desirable locations, as the ideal ones never agreed.

The concept added a completely new dimension to emergency care on highways, and the results exceeded our expectations. The number of lives saved was far higher than we had imagined or expected. Once a patient's vital functions were stabilized, the ambulance could safely transport them to the right hospital.

As the centers became operational, they quickly captured the public's attention.

People living nearby, including those from remote villages, started using these stations for their medical issues. This was an unexpected yet welcome fringe benefit. To support this, we stocked basic medicines, dressings, and supplies for common ailments.

To complete the system, we established a robust hospital network spanning from Kengeri to Mysore, covering key locations such as Bidadi, Ramanagara, Channapatna, Maddur, and Mandya. Mandya had the additional advantage of Sanjog Hospital and the Mandya Institute of Medical Sciences, ensuring advanced care when needed.

Once the highway emergency response project proved successful, word spread quickly. Many people came to observe the system in action, and several organizations offered their support. Among them was CAMHADD, an international NGO led by Dr. Pandurangi from Bristol, UK. During his visit, he presented the program to the World Health Organization (WHO), which subsequently decided to send a delegation to study it further.

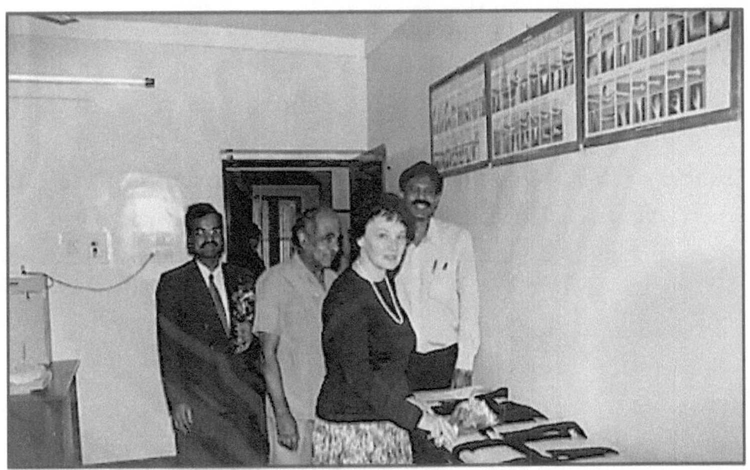

Miss Roberta Ritson Visiting Hoskote Centre

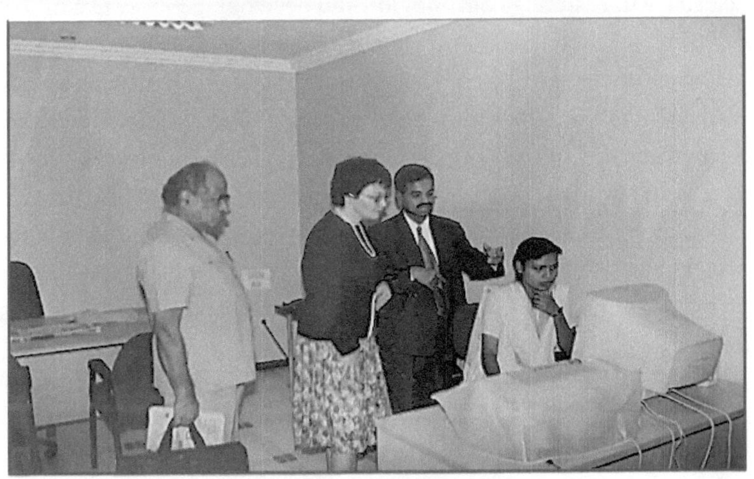

Visit of Miss Roberta Ritson to CTC Control Room

The WHO team was led by Dr. Roberta Ritson, who arrived in Bangalore for a week-long visit. During her stay, she conducted a comprehensive review of the entire system — visiting the central control room, observing its operations, and touring the Hosakote center, Indian Oil station at Narsapura, and Dabaspet. She also inspected the solar-powered first-aid centers, the mass-casualty response wagon, and several ambulances in service.

Dr. Ritson personally observed a few rescue operations and later compiled a detailed report, highlighting the program as a model for developing nations. Her appreciation and constructive feedback were deeply gratifying to all of us.

She also shared valuable insights from similar initiatives in other parts of the world, particularly in Africa and other developing regions, helping us refine and strengthen our own system.

Invitation to Geneva

A year later, we received an invitation to present the CTC model at Geneva. The program was exceptionally well-organized and warmly received.

Several international NGOs participated, and one day was dedicated exclusively to fostering collaboration and developing innovative models of community-based healthcare and emergency response.

During the event, I had a special meeting with Dr. Etienne Krug, Head of the Noncommunicable Diseases and Injury Prevention Division at the World Health Organization (WHO). Our discussion was detailed and thought-provoking, covering strategies to scale up the CTC model, explore adaptations for different contexts, and identify potential partnerships. While WHO did not offer direct financial support, they extended technical guidance, training materials, and expertise to help strengthen and expand the initiative.

Dr. Krug was particularly impressed with the CTC model, recognizing its potential relevance for developing countries. He even proposed exploring ways to implement and train similar systems in other nations. We agreed in principle, but the plan could not be fully realized. Nevertheless, the story and framework of the CTC model remain documented in WHO's records, a testament to its innovative approach and impact.

Building Lifelines Beyond Highways

Dr. Nandish, a popular surgeon from the Mandya Institute of Medical Sciences, was impressed by the project and took the initiative to create a mini trauma center at the medical college hospital.

Since he was at the helm of affairs from the institution's inception, he could create what was desirable. The entire emergency department was redesigned and upgraded. The facility was then inaugurated by the then Chief Minister, Sri H.D. Kumaraswamy.

Later, with the help of the college and the IMA (Indian Medical Association), several CMEs (Continuing Medical Education programs) were conducted in Mandya to educate doctors in the area.

A similar life-saving facility was set up at Ramanagar, in collaboration with Rotary Hospital.

With the support of the Rotary team and TTK Blood Bank, we created a temporary blood storage unit, a first of its kind for this stretch of the highway. Dr. Latha played a pivotal role in making this possible, taking a personal interest in the entire process. Her husband, a noted philanthropist, also extended tremendous support. TTK Blood Bank provided all the specialized equipment required for this initiative.

Beyond creating the storage facility, the organization took a step further and started providing free blood and plasma of all blood types. They were stocked on a consignment basis, and the availability of different blood groups was updated daily. They were also promptly replenished. To strengthen this setup, a blood group testing facility was also established at Rotary Hospital, Ramanagar. Until then, there was no way to access blood for emergencies before reaching Bangalore, which posed a serious risk to trauma patients. This new system changed everything. The outcome was overwhelming. Countless lives were saved because blood was available right when it was needed the most, in that critical golden window where minutes make the difference between life and death.

There were articles written about this in the media. More people became aware of our initiatives and offered their assistance. Sri Anantha Kumar MP, South Bangalore, donated an ambulance from MP Lad's funds.

Similarly, Sri DK Adhikesavulu also donated two ambulances, and he shared his ambition to extend similar highway care up to Chittoor in Andhra Pradesh.

For that, we sought the assistance of KSRTC and recreated a similar system, with ambulances stationed at Hosakote, extending all the way to Chittoor.

The community response was heartwarming. Many individuals came forward to offer space for parking ambulances, while others contributed to their upkeep. One petrol station owner in Palamaner even provided free fuel as his personal contribution to the cause.

Interestingly, these ambulances served more than just accident victims. They became a lifeline for rural communities. People from nearby villages used them to reach medical facilities for emergencies, including expectant mothers.

In fact, many pregnant women were safely transported for delivery, and at times, babies were delivered inside the ambulance itself.

This changed the game for us. It meant that our paramedic training had to be expanded beyond trauma care to include medical, respiratory, obstetric, and pediatric emergencies. We quickly wrote a new manual for managing these situations, and the ambulances were equipped with the necessary tools and medications to handle them. There was a significant reduction in mortality and disability rates. The sense of satisfaction in knowing that these interventions saved lives that might otherwise have been lost was truly immeasurable for us.

What began as an effort to respond to accidents gradually grew into a lifeline for entire communities. A way to support trauma victims, rural families, expectant mothers, and countless others in moments of dire need. These initiatives showed that highways are not just roads connecting cities, but pathways of responsibility, demanding preparedness, discipline, and care.

CHAPTER -7

Seven Hills & Sixty million Pilgrims : TTD-Sanjeevini

Pilgrimage is not just a trip that one takes for recreation. It is an extremely personal path of faith and renewal. People are also looking to redeem themselves. These paths are a sacred opportunity to heal, reflect and reconnect with a power that is probably greater than themselves. It is about finding peace and contentment. However, how does one cope when this sacred journey brings with it pain and tragedy instead of uplifting the soul.

I vividly remember my visit to Tirumala, one of the most revered pilgrimage sites for South Indians, when a sudden commotion erupted in the queue complex. I was standing a little away from the commotion, so I couldn't see what was the cause of it. From the whispers that were spreading quickly around, I deduced that a woman had slipped and fallen and was lying there injured, unable to get up. Everyone was trying to help her get up, but realized that she had injured her knee to do that. So, people started calling for help. In 15 to 20 minutes, the TTD staff arrived. However, due to the huge crowd and the numerous stairs and routes, they had to struggle to reach the patient and get her out, opening many barricades along the way.

This was not an isolated incident. With the massive crowds, the steep hills to climb, and the seemingly endless queues, medical emergencies in Tirumala were far more frequent than most people realize. The tragedy is that, in such conditions, getting timely help becomes nearly impossible. It felt wrong that people who come here seeking peace and divine solace are instead exposed to suffering and risk. After witnessing the incident, I felt compelled to take action.

Once I completed the darshan with my family, I went straight to meet the Executive Officer (EO) of the temple.

By then, however, he had left for the day. Fortunately, the staff was considerate and connected me to him over the phone. The EO, Mr. Ajeya Kallam, IAS, responded graciously and invited me to meet him at his home office at 2:30 p.m. During our meeting, I explained to him the scene I had witnessed and expressed my intention of establishing an emergency service for the temple to prevent such incidents from happening in the future. I also explained to him the kind of work being done at Bangalore by CTC, so that he could understand how efficient the system is. He was happy after hearing my idea and asked me to give a formal proposal. Thus, the idea of creating a service not only to the temple but to the entire 7 hills was born.

From my medical college days, I had often heard about the medical challenges at Tirumala. Managing such a massive influx of devotees every single day, and even more during special occasions, was nothing short of a Herculean task. I have extremely graphic memories of a few tragic bus accidents on the ghat road leading to the temple. Tirumala's roads make the journey a threatening challenge, due to steep and winding roads. Another problem that arises is the high altitude. Three thousand and eighty feet makes breathing extremely difficult for the pilgrims who are majorly the elderly. Medical issues like vomiting and nausea because of the serpentine bends, dehydration, and other travel-related problems occurred frequently. Fortunately, after the opening of the second ghat road, many of these incidents reduced significantly. We proposed a plan to position ambulances at strategic points, set up first-aid facilities within the temple premises, and train temple staff in basic emergency care. Several rounds of meetings were held with the TTD staff, and while everyone agreed on the urgency and importance of the initiative, the actual steps toward implementation moved slowly.

During this process, Mr. Ajeya Kallam was transferred. By the time the new EO, Mr. Sharma, took over, we had lost several months. But we weren't sitting idle during those months. We began gathering ambulances with the support of generous well-wishers. Mr. Syamaraju of Divyasree and Mr. Jeetu of the Embassy came forward to contribute, followed by Mr. D.K. Adikeasavulu Naidu, who added two more vehicles.

Finally, Tirupati MLA Mr. Venkataramana also joined hands by donating two vehicles. Altogether, we had five ambulances, which were proudly branded as TTD–Sanjeevini.

By then, it was time for Brahmotsavam, the nine-day annual festival at the Sri Venkateswara Temple in Tirumala, dedicated to Lord Venkateswara. Preparations had already begun in order to manage the massive number of devotees.

To handle the situation, multiple meetings were held. However, despite all this, medical arrangements were not prioritised enough. We decided to move forward and implement our system. Since we were ready, the very least we could do is be ready to provide crucial support throughout the festival. We drove down all our vehicles and parked them at the EO's office, formally requesting him to authorize the program.

He immediately called for an emergency meeting with all the medical institutions in Tirupati. Most of them insisted they were already well-prepared and showed reluctance to change the system. At that point, the EO decisively took control. He issued clear orders that CTC would implement the program and that every institution must provide its full support, without exception.

To mark the beginning, he organized a small press meet, performed a pooja for the vehicles, and officially inaugurated the service in October 2005. Over the next two days, we stayed to design and implement the entire system. After the inauguration, everyone became cooperative, so that by the next three days, the whole system was up and running.

1. Ambulances equipped: All the ambulances were fully equipped and made ready for deployment.

2. Seamless communication: TTD had its own dedicated wireless network that connected Tirupati and Tirumala. The same system was installed and connected to the ambulances, making it an integral part of their existing network, thereby ensuring smooth and reliable communication.

3. Strategic placement of ambulances: Vehicles were stationed at:

- No. 1 Choultry, Tirupati
- Alipiri foothills (where the two ghat roads meet)
- 36th turning (midway access point on the ghats)
- Mokali Parvatam
- In front of the main temple

4. First-aid centers were created: Emergency aid units were established at strategic locations, each equipped with first-aid kits and spine boards.

- Gali Gopuram
- Deer Park near the Hanuman statue
- The queue complexes
- Inside the temple near Kalyana Utsava Mandapam

5. Central control room: A control room was established at the Alipiri toll gate for all communication, monitoring, and coordination purposes.

6. Hospital network integration: Depending on the emergency, patients were transferred to Aswini Hospital (Tirumala), SVRR, SVIMS, or BIRD Hospital (Tirupati). Later, services were extended up to Alamelu Mangapuram.

We also provided basic first-aid training to key TTD staff, enabling them to step in whenever required, especially within the main temple, where rescuing a patient can be extremely challenging. By utilizing training, they were able to pick up the best ways to respond correctly and safely in emergency situations.

Once the system was stable and in place, the Brahmotsavam began, each and every medical emergency was quickly attended to. There was a noticeable improvement in the quality of care due to the number of rescues increasing rapidly.

Many devotees expressed their gratitude, and we received an outpouring of positive feedback. The service continued successfully for almost ten years, with TTD extending full support, including the maintenance of ambulances.

To ensure smooth functioning, Mr. Hanumantha Rao was appointed by CTC as the full-time manager. With remarkable dedication, he oversaw operations, coordinated staff, and made sure the services ran efficiently.

Mass Casualty Management

Mass casualties are every responder's worst nightmare. Not only because of the large number of victims, but also due to the severity and complexity of their injuries. After managing the highway system for a few years, we faced several such incidents. In an event where multiple people are injured simultaneously; the challenges increase drastically. These unfortunate events often occur in locations that are difficult to access. Providing medical assistance or social support becomes a challenge. The volume of resources needed to ensure an effective response time is something that cannot be fathomed. In such situations, there is a limitation of support. The most critical task becomes prioritizing and deciding who needs immediate attention and care. This is done to ensure that as many lives as possible are saved.

Normally, those who are at high risk of death will be taken to the ambulance and treated first. However, this often led to chaos. Others, who had to wait, felt that they were delayed or neglected. We even witnessed fights breaking out at ambulance rescue points, as everyone wanted to be taken first, regardless of their condition. With only one ambulance available, which can carry just two patients at a time, the situation became a nightmare for both us and the system. In addition, managing a mass casualty is altogether a different ball game. The maximum we could initially do was to summon more ambulances through the wireless network. However, uncertainties remain about availability and the ability to reach in time. So, transportation was a major challenge.

The second biggest challenge was at the hospitals themselves. Though most had emergency departments, they were far from being adequately equipped to handle mass casualties. Each time such an incident occurred, chaos ensued. Staff and attendants became confused, people ran helter-skelter trying to organize stretchers, oxygen, or basic supplies, and there was no structured system in place to direct the flow of patients. The lack of preparedness only magnified the crisis. It was a great eye-opener and a profound learning experience for us.

The third challenge was mobilizing resources in real-time, whether it involved arranging sufficient medical supplies, coordinating blood, or assembling a team of doctors on short notice. In emergencies of such scale, every single minute matters, and the delay in pooling manpower and material often becomes a race against time.

We were extremely set on being able to amend this. The initial step would be to diligently study pre-existing methodologies created for managing mass casualties. I made sure to personally look through protocols and rules followed in regions that are repeatedly hit by natural calamities. This included Japan and Indonesia, as well as civilian systems from other parts of the globe. We also approached the World Health Organization (WHO) for aid and guidance.

These insights became the foundation for a new system. Eventually, in collaboration with the WHO and Rajiv Gandhi University, we developed a comprehensive Mass Casualty Management Protocol. It was practical, systematic, and adaptable to our local needs.

This was one of the largest exercises we undertook across Bangalore city. We began with extensive data collection from every hospital, covering details such as bed strength, infrastructure, specialties, and super-specialties available, whether specialists were full-time or part-time, technology and equipment, laboratory and diagnostic services, pharmacy support, mortuary facilities, and every other resource that could play a role in emergency management.

According to international standards, 7–10% of hospital beds must be reserved for mass casualty situations. Unfortunately, our emergency infrastructure was so poorly planned that hardly any hospital could meet this requirement. Yet, instead of being discouraged, we designed a protocol tailored to our local circumstances. This protocol clearly defined the role and responsibility of each individual in the system, ensuring that when a crisis struck, there would be no confusion, no overlap, and no crisscrossing of efforts.

Rescue Wagon

To overcome the challenges of transporting mass casualty accident victims safely, we introduced the concept of converting a bus into a Rescue Wagon to the Karnataka State Road Transport Corporation (KSRTC). This collaboration deepened our partnership with KSRTC, expanding it across multiple dimensions.

We trained all KSRTC drivers and conductors in first aid, supplied them with fully stocked first-aid kits, and equipped buses operating on highways with spine boards. Gradually, the entire crew became confident in handling emergencies. They knew what to do and, more importantly, what not to do. At the time, Mr. Bhaskar Rao, IPS, served as the Managing Director of KSRTC. A man deeply passionate about accident prevention, he conducted extensive research on the Bangalore–Mysore Highway, identifying accident-prone zones and developing systematic recommendations to reduce mishaps.

Chief Engineer Mr. Mukkanna took up the project of the rescue wagon with great enthusiasm and personally oversaw the design and development, securing approvals and initiating the build. I made frequent visits to monitor progress, and together we built a highly functional prototype, the first of its kind in the country.

The Rescue Wagon was formally inaugurated by the hon'ble Chief minister Sri H.D. Kumaraswamy, who personally inspected the vehicle and its facilities. The wagon could transport up to 16 patients simultaneously, providing comprehensive medical support en route to the hospital. It was designed as a self-contained emergency unit, equipped to handle all stages of care from rescue and resuscitation to first aid, treatment initiation, and continuous monitoring.

Key features included:

- Capacity to rescue 8 critically injured and 8–10 walking wounded at once.
- Stretchers with safety straps, IV fluid support, oxygen supply, suction units, and vital sign monitors.
- Spine boards, neck stabilizers, and oxygen masks for trauma care.

- Under-seat storage for emergency dressings, antiseptics, essential medicines, and intravenous fluids.
- Automated External Defibrillator (AED) to record ECG, interpret cardiac rhythm, and treat cardiac arrest.
- Two-way communication systems connecting hospitals and police.
- Digital interfaces enabling real-time medical guidance from the central control room during rescue and resuscitation.
- Two jumbo oxygen cylinders, multiple first-aid kits, ladders, and complete extrication tools for difficult rescues.
- Staffed by trained paramedics, ready to initiate treatment and maintain monitoring throughout transport.

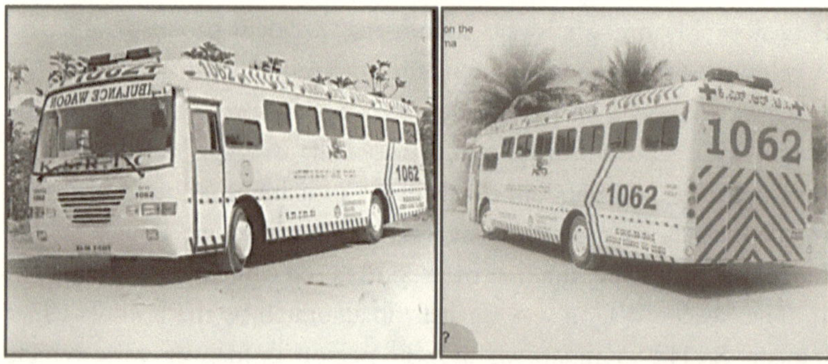

Mass Casualty Rescue Wagon

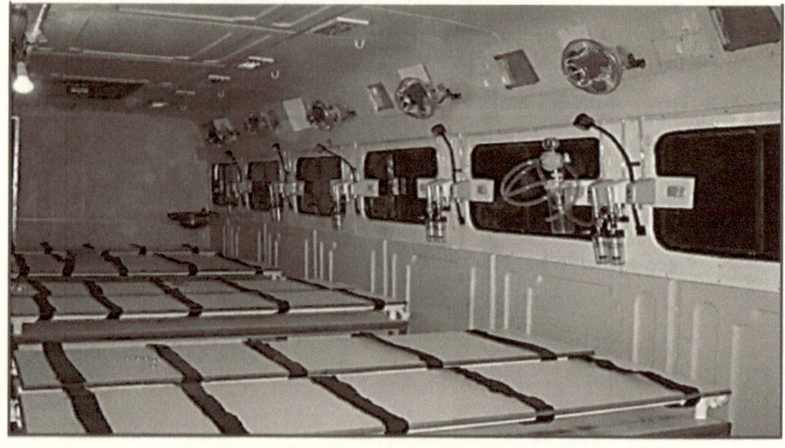

Interiors of the Wagon

Over time, as maintenance challenges emerged, the vehicle's use became less frequent.

However, after repairs and refurbishing, it was re-dedicated to the public on 10th September by Hon. Minister for Transport Sri Ramalinga Reddy, in the presence of Sri Umashankar (MD, KSRTC) and Sri Sunder Raju (MD, Atria Group).

At its peak, the Rescue Wagon proved to be a boon to the public, performing service during several emergencies. It was deployed not only on highways around Bangalore but also during the Coorg floods and landslides, as well as the Kerala floods, providing timely medical rescue and relief.

Commitment and Discipline: The Missing Links in Our Emergency Response

In a mass casualty situation, protocols and guidelines alone cannot save lives. While everything may appear easy and straight to the point on paper, it is not that way in reality. Follow instructions, stay calm, let the trained responders do their job. It is not so simple. To put together a successful rescue operation, everything depends on the mindset of the people who are involved. Once tragedy strikes, sense goes out of the window, and panic takes over. People often ignore the instructions that could save their lives. They rush and run about, resulting in more harm than escape.

What should have been a coordinated response quickly turns into chaos, with fear spreading from one person to another until even a manageable situation spirals out of control.

This is why massive casualties are not only a medical problem but a social fact. Discipline, trust, and commitment are just as important as any equipment or training. A mass casualty response works like a chain, with rescuers, systems, and the public as its links. The whole chain will collapse if even one link breaks, like when people are unable to cooperate. This is the reason behind the different ways in which countries handle crises. Some display impeccable efficiency and others struggle to keep up. While in some cases there may be similar resources and rules in place, the results are often very different.

It is not due to technological inconsistencies but multiple other factors. This includes culture, discipline, and the ability of individuals to prioritize collective survival over individual fears. Look at the Indian crowd, for example; our lack of civic sense and the desire to save ourselves first often lead to stampedes and crowding, resulting in a commotion so intense that no rescuers can work properly. Even during an accident, onlookers crowd the scene in their desire to witness and capture the scene on their mobiles, while the rescuers have to push their way to the accident site. Getting out after pushing away all the crowd is even more difficult.

I happened to be in Japan last year, in 2024, when the tragic aircraft accident took place at Haneda Airport. A flight from Sapporo to Tokyo carrying 379 passengers collided with a Japan Coast Guard aircraft right on the runway.

Both planes immediately caught fire and were reduced to ashes. Yet, in an extraordinary feat, every single passenger was rescued safely within 90 seconds. This was a task that only a country like Japan could accomplish.

The incident was televised and broadcast worldwide. While thousands of people watch with their breath held, I truly wonder how many are able to realize the amount of preparation, discipline, and training that goes into successfully executing a rescue. I have visited multiple countries and met multiple people. There is one distinct observation that I have made. The Japanese stand out in their commitment to health care.

Coincidentally, I was in Japan and was able to witness the rescue effort very closely. This opportunity gave me the chance to genuinely appreciate the effort and perseverance that went into it. Each individual acted with utmost commitment and pure skill.

There was no pandemonium, chaos or uncertainty. The crew had already been trained tediously before getting into the field. They already knew exactly what to do and made sure to do it swiftly. The system on the field worked precisely, and each step fell into its place.

And perhaps most impressive of all were the passengers themselves, who followed every instruction calmly, without panic, and without moving from their respective places, trusting the process and allowing the rescue to unfold smoothly. This is an emphasis on the general discipline of the people in the country, without which the rescue would have been a nightmare. Imagine people running around, crying, pushing each other aside in a rush to get outside, and fights breaking out with the crew and passengers.

No matter how much the crew knew about the perfect evacuation plan, all those skills would go to waste unless it is executed in the right way. This is exactly why we say there is a difference between knowing the rules in theory and actually practicing them in the moment of crisis. Commitment and precision are what make the real difference. The way the pilots, crew, ground rescue teams, and all the support services responded was impeccable.

Their readiness to act, make decisions, and execute in a professional manner was clearly visible.

Equally remarkable was the precision. If you observe closely, every decision taken, every order given, every announcement made followed one another instantly, without argument, hesitation, or delay. Everyone knew their role and carried it out exactly as expected. There was no confusion, no overlap, no crisscrossing.

This is the reason behind the safe rescue of 379 passengers in a mere 90 seconds. This incident runs deeper than just being a story of victory or lives being heroically saved. It was an example of how both individual and collective skills can make a difference. This rescue operation serves as a testament to what disaster management should truly be.

The years of training and practice the crew received through countless dummy drills and simulations, as well as rehearsing every possible scenario until it became second nature, are truly appreciated. Such preparation does not happen overnight. It is the result of well-designed protocols, precise processes, and repeated practice, combined with a deep commitment to their profession.

It was also a reminder that such results are never the work of one person alone. It was a collective effort where every individual, from pilots to ground staff, knew their role and played it with discipline.

Without that shared commitment and unity, no system, no matter how advanced, could achieve this level of efficiency. This is the uniqueness of Japan: a culture where discipline, training, and professionalism converge to turn the impossible into reality. It is a quality we must admire and, more importantly, strive to emulate.

Everyone must at least know the basics of how to deal with emergencies. Forget the large-scale disasters and think about the day-to-day life accidents we witness. We see so many incidents that could have been avoided with a little awareness. Yet, the level of ignorance we face is staggering.

It is not impossible to build efficient systems; in fact, the technical part is often the easiest. What we lack are core values such as commitment, discipline, and honesty.

Too often, everyone wants to play commander.

Nobody wants to follow instructions, and instead of cooperation, we create confusion. As a result, even simple situations become complicated and chaotic. The lack of discipline of our citizens is glaring. Instead of helping a system run smoothly, people disrupt it with suspicion, insecurity, and incompetence. The only way forward is serious, systematic training that must be introduced across every sector. Even in the medical field, where numerous effective systems exist, there is still a long way to go before we achieve excellence.

We must be willing to learn from countries like Japan, where discipline and preparation are ingrained in the culture. Only then can we truly claim to be a developed nation.

CHAPTER – 8

Towards a National Golden Hour Network

L ife-Saving Measures: What Everyone Must Know
Golden hour is the first hour after an injury. Generally, the accident or injury is the primary event and lasts not more than a few seconds. However, a series of complications often ensues after that. They include bleeding, vomiting, convulsions or fits, shock, breathing difficulty, lack of oxygen to the body, and tissue swelling. The majority of such problems occur within the first hour after the accident. These secondary problems will complicate the original injury and are most often the cause of death and disability. Moreover, when a person is unconscious, they can't take care of themselves. They all require immediate medical attention and assistance. If there are no secondary complications, it will result in a better outcome. It may sound difficult, but with an effective system, we can avoid all the secondary complications.

Effective treatment in the Golden Hour can reduce:
- Immediate death
- Immediate and permanent disability
- Reduce complications
- Reduce ICU stay
- Reduce the time of hospitalization.
- Reduce the medical costs.
- Improve the quality of survival.

1. Secondary Changes

After the primary impact, the body undergoes a series of secondary changes. These are direct consequences of the original injury and usually occur within the first hour or two. The injured person may lose consciousness, suffer heavy bleeding externally or internally, experience convulsions or fits, or develop swelling at the injury site. Swelling on the face, in particular, can block the airway and lead to breathing difficulties. Some may even drown in their own secretions or vomit, which is a frequent occurrence. Shock or spinal injuries are also common. It is essential to recognize these secondary problems because most of them are preventable. If neglected, however, they can aggravate the original injury and lead to life-threatening complications.

2. ABCDE

ABCDE stands for Airway, Breathing, Circulation, Disability or Neurological Deficits, and Exposure. These are as fundamental to life as the alphabet is to learning. Any compromise in them can quickly become life-threatening. That is why recognizing and addressing them without delay is so important. The moment you detect a problem, seek urgent medical help by calling an ambulance, alerting a paramedic, or rushing to the nearest hospital. If trained, initiate CPR immediately. These simple, timely actions often make the difference between life and death.

3. Bleeding

Bleeding is one of the most dangerous and life-threatening complications after an injury. The warning signs are often subtle, like a weak pulse, falling blood pressure, rapid breathing as if gasping for air, or sudden confusion. When there is an external injury, it is visible to the naked eye and can be identified swiftly. Internal bleeding however, raised many more red flags. It is dangerous and deceptive. There may be no external wound but internally there may be severe damage. Since it takes so long to recognize, situations often become critical.

4. Spine Injury

The spine connects the brain and the body through an extensive network of nerve fibers. Spine injury can occur in all high-speed injuries, falls from great heights, and also in high-impact injuries.

Spine injuries are often not visible from the outside unless you take an X-ray. When it comes to the spine, the neck bones are the most vulnerable because of their mobility, followed by the lower back and trunk. That is why every unconscious person must be treated as a potential spine injury case until proven otherwise. The same applies if someone complains of pain along the spine or shows weakness or difficulty moving their hands or legs. In such situations, never move them carelessly. The spine must be immobilized, and shifting should only be done with proper assistance to avoid worsening the injury.

5. Fracture

Persistent pain, deformity of the hand or leg, loss of movement, and pain increasing on attempted movement are the common indicators of a fracture. X-ray examination can diagnose it accurately. Inadvertent movement can cause complete dislocation of the bone or joints, and the bone fragments can protrude from the skin, making it a compound fracture. More importantly, the adjacent blood vessel or nerve can be cut by the fractured bones, causing serious injury to the leg or hand. This is why it is important to immobilize the limb when a fracture is suspected.

6. Mobilization

Many problems can happen while shifting an injured individual. Improper shifting can worsen the spinal injury or dislodge a clot. This is extremely dangerous as it can cause unexpected sudden bleeding. In some scenarios, it can further dislocate an already existing fracture. Hence, proper transportation is necessary. It must also include appropriate assistance, equipment, and trained personnel.

Universal Recovery Position

The recovery position is a simple yet lifesaving technique used when a person is unresponsive but breathing normally with a steady pulse. Placing someone in this position helps to keep their airway open, allows fluids such as saliva, vomit, or blood to drain safely, and prevents choking or aspiration. It also maintains the body in a stable posture until professional help arrives.

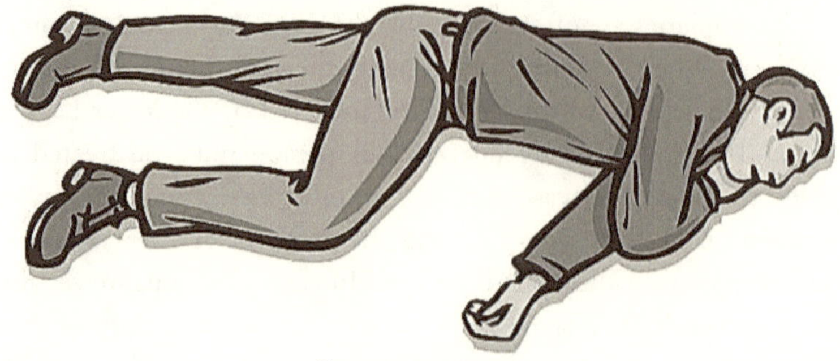

Recovery position

The universal recovery position can be safely applied to people of all ages and in almost all emergency situations. The procedure involves:

- Kneel by the injured and straighten their legs.
- If they are wearing glasses or have any bulky items in their pockets, remove them.
- Do not search their pockets for small items.
- Place the arm that is nearest to you at a right angle to their body, with the elbow bent and their palm facing upwards.
- Bring their other arm across their chest and place the back of their hand against the cheek nearest to you. Hold it there.
- With your other hand, pull their far knee up so that their foot is flat on the floor.
- Keeping the back of the injured hand pressed against their cheek, pull on the far leg to roll the person towards you onto their side. You can then adjust the top leg so that it is bent at a right angle.
- Gently tilt the person's head back and lift their chin to ensure their airway remains open. You can adjust the hand under their cheek to do this.

This simple position can make the difference between life and death, as it protects an unconscious person's airway and ensures they continue to breathe effectively while awaiting medical attention.

7. First Aid

This is one of the simplest yet most crucial life-saving measures, especially for anyone whose ABCDE is compromised. It must be started the very moment the need is recognized. While these steps may look simple, they require proper training and certification.

One must be both familiar and confident in applying them correctly because in such critical situations, a single mistake can make things worse instead of better.

CPR (Cardiopulmonary Resuscitation)

CPR is the first line of action when the airway, breathing, or circulation fails. If a person is not breathing or the heart has stopped pumping effectively, the brain can suffer irreversible damage within minutes, regardless of the original injury. Knowing how to perform CPR properly and administering it at the right time can mean the difference between life and death.

8. Transportation in an Ambulance

An ambulance is always the safest option while transporting a patient, rather than private vehicles with cramped space and less safety. However, it is never just about putting someone into an ambulance. Safe transportation is a science in its own right. It means moving the patient at the right time during the golden hour, to the right place where definitive treatment is available, handled by the right people, like trained paramedics, using the right methods of shifting, monitoring, and care. To make this possible, the ambulance must be more than a vehicle; it must be a mobile emergency unit. It should always be equipped with essential tools, including a proper First Aid kit, spine board, neck collar, AED (Automated External Defibrillator), oxygen supply, and emergency medications for shock and pain relief.

9. Role of a Paramedic

A paramedic is the one who is adequately trained in the use of all equipment in the ambulance, administers medications, starts an intravenous line, and monitors vital signs throughout the journey. Additionally, he can rescue, resuscitate, identify life-threatening situations, act appropriately, and communicate with the hospital in advance to ensure seamless continuity of treatment.

A Good Samaritan

Any citizen who takes the responsibility of helping the injured at the scene is called a Good Samaritan. Their role can be significant apart from life-saving. The roles they can play are many. The important ones are:

- Shift the injured to a safe place
- Call for an ambulance
- Protect the belongings
- Avoid the crowding of mobs
- Check ABCDE if known
- Administer first aid and CPR if trained
- Inform the friends or relatives
- Assist in transportation to the hospital
- ✓ **Do's:** Everyone should come forward to help the victims of accidents. Follow the steps mentioned earlier and, in addition, offer extra assistance wherever it is safe and appropriate. Remember, in emergencies, genuine help is never penalized by the police or anyone else.
- ✗ **Don'ts:** Never leave an injured person unattended. Do not pour water into the mouth of someone unconscious, and never attempt to shift a patient without proper assistance or support. Wrong handling can worsen the injury.

Ask for Help: Never hesitate to ask for help. Utilize any available local resources, such as people, vehicles, or other means. Human support and quick action at the scene often make all the difference.

Mass Casualties

If multiple people are affected either in an accident or in a natural calamity, the situation is called a mass casualty. It often occurs at unusual times and in unusual locations. Here, everyone, including the government, must act immediately.

Dealing with a mass casualty is a totally different ball game. Golden Hour has prepared a protocol defining the roles and responsibilities of the onlookers, ambulances, paramedics, and hospitals.

What to look out for?

1. How to Suspect Brain Injury

Any person who is unconscious or has even briefly lost consciousness must be treated as a possible case of brain injury. It is always safer to over-suspect until a medical professional rule it out, rather than take things lightly. Never assume the cause to be alcohol, medications, or fatigue. Such assumptions can delay the right care and cost a life.

2. How to Suspect Spinal Injury

If anyone complains of neck or back pain, has difficulty moving the spine, or shows signs of nerve-related problems, such as weakness, numbness, or loss of movement in the arms or legs, spinal injury must be suspected in every unconscious person and ruled out only after a proper X-ray or scan. In any case, it is safer to immobilize the neck and shift with a spinal board till injury is excluded in the hospital. Most of the time, a spine injury is a hidden injury. Only an X-ray or CT/MRI scan can exclude the possibility. Shifting such people inadvertently can damage the spinal cord and produce permanent paralysis. With proper precautions, such a calamity can be avoided.

3. How to Suspect Bleeding

Reduction in pulse volume or BP, air hunger, vomiting of blood, breathlessness, and confusion are the common signs of bleeding. External bleeding can be visible, but internal bleeding is not. The common sites for bleeding are the chest, abdomen, pelvis, and fractures of long bones. In children, even the scalp can bleed torrentially. They require immediate first aid and rapid transportation to the appropriate hospital. Paramedics, meanwhile, should support with all available measures. Otherwise, shock can ensue, leading to a life-threatening situation as well as brain damage.

Who Needs Hospitalization?

- Anyone who is unconscious, even briefly
- Any kind of bleeding, external or suspected internal
- Fits (seizures) or repeated vomiting

- Presence of neurological problems such as weakness, numbness, or loss of movement
- High-velocity injuries, including road accidents or falls from height
- Children and the elderly, even if injuries seem minor
- Whenever there is doubt or suspicion, it is always safer to get checked.

Things to Remember

Accidents are best avoided, but if they occur, the key is to act quickly and correctly. Always focus on doing the first, most important steps without hesitation. Learn to anticipate danger and spot problems before they worsen. Never assume things will be fine on their own. In real life circumstances, everything that can go wrong will probably end up going south. On top of that, it will happen at the worst possible moment.

Educate Others

It is important to learn first aid and CPR for critical moments that can come up at any time. You need to be able to make a difference. By taking the initiative to enroll yourself in certified courses, you provide yourself with the opportunity to act quickly during emergencies. Actively volunteering helps you put your skills into effect. Spreading your knowledge with others helps you understand what you picked up and also ensures more people are able to respond in a timely manner.

It is more than spreading awareness, it is about creating a continuous system that incorporates safety and care. One day it maybe remembered as a lifesaver.

Self-Discipline

Prevention of accidents begins with self-discipline and constant attentiveness. Qualities that must be cultivated even before obtaining a driving license. Driving should never be approached casually, and it is important to correct unsafe behavior in others as well.

Also, your mental state plays a crucial role in driving and accidents. Avoid driving when you are upset, agitated, or distracted.

It is always better to pause than to risk lives and regret later. Good health and physical fitness further support safe driving practices. By embracing responsibility and changing our attitude toward road safety, we can transform the culture and make Indian roads truly safe.

Road Rage

Road rage is on the rise, and it poses a serious threat to everyone's safety. Aggressive behavior on the roads, whether directed at other drivers or pedestrians, only escalates tension and leads to harmful consequences. Choosing to remain calm and composed can defuse many situations that might otherwise spiral out of control. Shouting, making offensive gestures, or engaging in fights is unnecessary and dangerous. If we all make the effort to start our journeys on time, follow traffic rules, and behave in a civilized manner, countless instances of road rage and accidents can be prevented.

Privileged Vehicles

Emergency vehicles like Police cars, Fire trucks, and Ambulances hold extraordinary privileges on the road because they serve critical purposes such as security, safety, and life-saving, respectively. Their sirens are not just loud sounds but vital signals alerting everyone to make way immediately. Among them, an ambulance carries the highest urgency, as every minute can decide between life and death for a patient in critical condition.

Giving way to ambulances is not just a rule but a moral responsibility. At the same time, ambulance drivers must be well-trained to handle high-pressure situations, drive safely at special speeds, and provide first aid or assist in rescues when required.

These privileges should never be misused; rather, they should be exercised with efficiency, responsibility, and respect for the lives they are entrusted to protect.

Above all, ambulances can have some special rights:

- To travel right off the way
- To jump the signal, if necessary
- To move in a one-way street to cut short the distance

- To park even in the middle of the road in order to rescue an individual in an emergency
- To overtake and to go beyond the notified speed limits when necessary

However, all these measures must be implemented within safe limits and without causing harm to other road users.

As far as the public is concerned, the moment they hear the siren of the ambulance, they are supposed to pull their vehicle to the side and stay put till the ambulance moves ahead of them. One should not block the ambulance or chase the ambulance from behind to take advantage.

Generally, VIPs get such a preference in our country. Ambulances must be treated with much higher priority, for "VIP" means "Very Injured Person".

In the end, saving lives during the Golden Hour is not the responsibility of doctors and paramedics alone, it is a collective duty. Each one of us, as citizens, has a role to play: from preventing accidents through discipline to acting swiftly and sensibly when emergencies occur. Systems, technology, and ambulances can only work if people cooperate and respect their purpose.

Giving way to an ambulance, knowing basic first aid, and staying calm in a crisis are simple actions that carry immense power. If we all adopt these practices, our roads will not just be safer, they will become pathways of survival and hope.

In their Words

We met by accident.

(Orchestrated by Him).

I hear a siren blare.

I look into the rearview mirror.

It's an ambulance.

I pull over and let it pass.

The white ambulance with stripes, with the letters 'Operation Sanjeevini, ' zips past.

If the accident victim in the ambulance reaches a hospital and is provided trauma care within the golden hour, I know his chances of survival are high.

I feel a lump in my throat.

I know he will.

And I know I have also played a very, very small role in this.

Cut to Chennai.

Dr. Sharan Srinivasan, a junior to Dr. NKV and I are in conversation with the founders of Trauma Care Consortium. TCC was doing a fund-raising show with actor Kamal Hasan and I was chosen to be the anchor. Post my return to Bangalore, I mentioned to Sharan about TCC, and he introduced me to Dr. NKV, who was also on the threshold of launching CTC.

My humble role in the launch of CTC was organizing a press conference. The press gave us a fairly good coverage. And CTC grew in strength.

The success of this project apart from the support of service organizations and corporates was the involvement of Dr. NKV. His passion, the time, the effort, the commitment, the perseverance and above all, the conviction to make it a success was the sole reason for the success of CTC. And when there is sincerity of purpose, the cosmos aligns itself and energy flows.

It came in the form of Jagdish, Raj, SA Chandran, and many others. We are all good friends today, thanks to CTC.

When I look back today, I believe every act of ours comes with a purpose. My meeting with Dr. NKV and being a small supporting 'extra' in the CTC script was scripted by God.

I am thankful to Him.

- R T Kumar

Owner of Oysters advertising agency

Dial 1062: The Experience That Shaped My Life in Medicine

- Dr. Pramodh R K

Lifestyle Medicine, Perinatal Medicine & Addiction Medicine Physician

For many doctors, the early years of their career are filled with learning, long hours, and the pursuit of confidence in clinical decision-making.

But for me, those years became something far greater — a journey of purpose, mentorship, and service that shaped my entire outlook on medicine and humanity. From 2004 to 2010, as a young and passionate doctor, I served as the Chief Medical Officer at an Emergency Medical Centre affiliated with CTC Sanjeevini – Comprehensive Trauma Consortium.

This initiative, led by the visionary Dr. N. K. Venkataramana, was nothing short of groundbreaking — it introduced India's first-ever free ambulance service, known as CTC Sanjeevini Dial 1062, in Bengaluru.

Working under Dr. Venkataramana was an amazing experience. It wasn't just about treating emergencies; it was about being part of a movement that gave people hope when every second counted.

Each day brought new challenges: trauma cases, medical emergencies, and critical transfers. Yet behind every emergency call was a story of resilience and teamwork.

As Chief Medical Officer, I led from the front, stabilizing patients, guiding response teams, and ensuring safe transfers to tertiary hospitals, all completely free of cost. The experience demanded both skill and heart, and it was here that I discovered the true essence of emergency medicine: swift action grounded in empathy.

Beyond the ambulance bays and trauma wards, my commitment extended to public safety at large-scale events. Serving as the Chief Medical Officer for the international singer Aerosmith's concert, as well as for numerous other events across Bengaluru, I orchestrated comprehensive medical preparedness for thousands of attendees, ensuring that every possible emergency scenario was anticipated and addressed with calm precision.

This journey also led me into medical education, where I became associated with PRIME, a respected training institute founded by Dr. Venkataramana. There, I dedicated myself to training young doctors, paramedics, and students in emergency response and trauma management, sharing the values of readiness, teamwork, and compassion that had become central to my own practice.

Looking back, I describe those years as truly transformative. "It was an incredible phase working with a visionary mentor, witnessing the impact of free emergency care, and realizing how leadership and compassion can truly save lives."

Today, the lessons I learned during those formative years continue to guide me as a physician, a leader, and a lifelong student of medicine.

My story stands as a reminder that great healthcare is built not only on knowledge and systems, but on vision, empathy, and the will to serve humanity beyond measure.

Dr. Pramodh R K is a senior medical professional with extensive experience in emergency and trauma medicine. A dedicated clinician and mentor, he has contributed to several public health initiatives and medical training programs. His work reflects a deep commitment to compassionate care, leadership, and the advancement of emergency medical services in India.

For a Better Tomorrow

Time is life.

When a life is hanging in the balance, every passing second is invaluable. Every helping gesture is hope. This simple truth has guided my entire journey and shaped everything I have tried to build. From the concept of the Golden Hour to the creation of the Comprehensive Trauma Consortium, and every initiative that followed.

I did not set out to write this book as a collection of theories. I wrote it because I have seen lives lost, and I have seen lives saved. The difference between the two, more often than not, was time. I have seen the helplessness in families when their loved ones could not be rescued quickly enough. I have also seen the gratitude in their eyes when timely care brought someone back from the brink of death. These moments are etched into me forever, have molded me into the man I am today, and are the reason I decided to share my experiences with you.

The Golden Hour is not just a medical concept to me; it is a mission. It is the core of everything I have done in my professional and social journey. The first sixty minutes after a traumatic injury are decisive. They are the difference between survival and death, between recovery and permanent disability. If proper care is given during this time and the airway is secured, bleeding controlled, and vital signs stabilized, the outcome is transformed. If this window is lost, even the best hospitals and the most advanced doctors cannot undo the damage. That is why I have fought tirelessly to make people, governments, and communities understand: **saving lives begins before the hospital.**

Looking back, I realize that much of my work has been about building bridges between knowledge and action, between what is possible and what is actually practiced. Our hospitals are capable, our doctors are skilled, but too often the patient never reaches them in time.

The true battlefields where precious lives are won and lost are on the roads, in transportation, communication, and discipline.

That is why I created systems, trained paramedics, established ambulance networks, and worked with governments.

And that is why I continue to write, speak, and advocate, because awareness must become second nature for each of us.

Accidents are preventable. This is the truth that I want every reader of this book to take away. Most accidents occur not because of fate, but due to negligence, such as poor roads, careless driving, rule violations, or a lack of preparedness. Even when an accident does occur, the damage can almost always be reduced if immediate, correct action is taken. The tools are simple, the knowledge is available, but what we lack is discipline, commitment, and the will to act responsibly.

My purpose in writing this book is very clear: to save lives. The suggestions and practices I have shared are not difficult. They do not require special training or great resources. They require only awareness, responsibility, and compassion. If each of us commits to following the simplest of safety precautions, if each of us respects the Golden Hour, the difference will be profound.

I have often been asked, 'how do we build a safer future?' The answer is straightforward. The future depends on education and culture. Adults often carry fixed mindsets, with habits that have been formed over the years. It is difficult to alter these unless they themselves experience or realize the dangers of negligence. We can create awareness, yes, but change must come from within. Fines and strict enforcement of the law are necessary, but they are temporary measures. Real transformation comes when culture changes. And that is why our children and youth hold the key.

Young minds are moldable. They are eager to learn and quick to adopt new practices. They are also far more aware of global standards than generations before them. I strongly believe that every school-going child should be taught about road safety, basic first aid, and emergency response. Just as they learn mathematics and science, they must learn the rules of survival and compassion. Imagine a society where every teenager knows how to help someone in distress without causing further harm, where every child grows up with the habit of following traffic rules as naturally as they learn to write their name.

That is the society that will save lives.

I have personally seen the difference such training can make. When we conducted programs in schools, training lakhs of students and teachers in Bangalore, the response was overwhelming. The change was visible. Children grew more confident, more responsible, and many even expressed interest in making this a career. If we can make such training part of the school curriculum, mandatory and systematic, the impact will be immeasurable.

The role of technology in the future cannot be overstated. The coming years hold exciting possibilities. Artificial intelligence, nanotechnology, biomolecular research, regenerative medicine, and advanced imaging will revolutionize the way we diagnose, treat, and prevent diseases. Emergency care will also be transformed with drones delivering medical kits, real-time tracking of ambulances, wearable devices that alert responders before a collapse, and AI systems predicting complications before they occur. These are not dreams for the distant future. They are already being developed.

But technology alone will not save lives. Technology is only as effective as the system that supports it and the people who use it. A well-equipped ambulance is useless if stuck in traffic without a clear path in front of it. A hospital with the best facilities cannot help if the patient never arrives on time. This is why discipline, awareness, and culture matter as much as innovation. The two must go hand in hand.

Think back to the aircraft accident in Japan, where discipline and training saved hundreds of lives in a mass casualty situation. The difference was not only in technology but also in the mindset of the people, including their commitment to following instructions, discipline in acting collectively, and precision in performing tasks without chaos. That is what we must learn and adopt. Without discipline, no matter how many protocols are in place, they will not succeed. I want these pages to be a reminder for each and every one of you. Saving lives is not the sole responsibility of doctors.

It is a shared responsibility of governments, institutions, communities, and most importantly, individuals. Each one of us can make a difference.

Giving way to an ambulance, following traffic rules, helping an injured person the right way, and spreading awareness; all of these can contribute to saving a life.

Do not treat this book as just words on a page. Treat it as a personal responsibility. Start with yourself. Wear your helmet, wear your seatbelt, drive responsibly. Teach your children the right practices. Support systems that promote emergency preparedness. Volunteer when possible. Be a Good Samaritan. If each one of us does even a fraction of this, the ripple effect will transform our society.

The road to change is never quick, but it is always worth it. Rome was not built in a day, and neither will a safe nation be. But every step, every act of responsibility, every moment of discipline moves us closer. The journey may be long, but the destination is worth every effort.

It has been 25 years since I started this journey. For me, the Golden Hour has never been just a theory. It is a lifeline. It is the bridge between tragedy and survival, between despair and hope. And it is within our reach, if only we choose to act.

So, I ask you, as I close this book: will you be part of the change? Will you take the responsibility to make our roads safer, our responses quicker, and our communities stronger? Will you commit to saving lives, even if it is just one?

Because sometimes, one life is everything.

About the Author

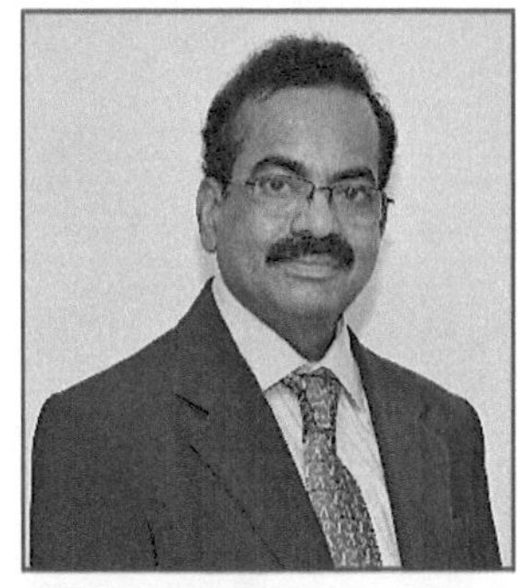

Dr. N.K. Venkataramana is a well-known neurosurgeon and founder Chairman of BRAINS Super Specialty Hospital, Bangalore. After his medical graduation from SV Medical college, Tirupati, did his masters in Neurosurgery at NIMHANS. He served as Assistant Professor of NIMHANS later established Manipal institute of neurological disorders, and BGS institute of Neurosciences. He had his micro neurosurgery and endoscopic neurosurgery training at Hannover and Mainz of Germany respectively.

He served at BGS Global Hospital as Vice Chairman. BRAINS is his brain child, a center of excellence offering comprehensive services for complex Brain and Spine disorders with a goal to set the gold standards in neuro care. He is instrumental in creating GPS based state of the art ambulance services for the Bangalore city, a first of its kind pre- hospital care system (1062). This is his social initiative in promoting social awareness of Golden Hours for head trauma and stroke.

He has 35 years of experience in neurosurgery with contributions to Endoscopic neurosurgery, Pediatric neurosurgery, Functional neurosurgery, Cerebrovascular surgery, Spine surgery and Stem cell research for brain and spine regeneration. He has several scientific publications and chapters in text books to his credit. He is a member of several national and international neurosurgical professional bodies and held several prestigious positions including the Editorship of Brain Voice, Journal of Cerebrovascular sciences and member of editorial board of many scientific journals. He had received many awards notably the Karnataka Rajyotsava Award from the state of Karnataka and Sir CV Raman centenary award from Honorable Prime Minister Shri Narendra Modi.